HEALTH PROMOTION

)07

8

HEALTH PROMOTION
Foundations for Practice

Jennie Naidoo

Senior Lecturer, Health Promotion,
University of the West of England, Bristol, UK

and

Jane Wills

Senior Lecturer, Health Promotion, South Bank University, London, UK

BAILLIÈRE TINDALL
London   Philadelphia   Toronto   Sydney   Tokyo

Baillière Tindall   24–28 Oval Road
W. B. Saunders   London NW1 7DX

The Curtis Center
Independence Square West
Philadelphia, PA 19106-3399, USA

Harcourt Brace & Company
55 Horner Avenue
Toronto, Ontario M8Z 4X6, Canada

Harcourt Brace & Company, Australia
30-52 Smidmore Street
Marrickville
NSW 2204, Australia

Harcourt Brace & Company, Japan
Ichibancho Central Building
22-1 Ichibancho
Chiyoda-ku , Tokyo 102, Japan

First published 1994
Second printing 1995

A catalogue record for this book is available from the British Library

ISBN 0-7020-1680-2

Typeset by Columns Design and Production Services Ltd, Reading
Printed and bound in Great Britain by Butler & Tanner Ltd, Frome and London

Contents

Publisher's Acknowledgements

Figure 1.2 a–e, from McKeown and Lowe, (1974), *An Introduction to Social Medicine*, reproduced with permission from Blackwell Scientific Publications, Oxford, UK.

Figure 3.1, from Andrews and Withey, (1976), *Social Indications of Well-being: American Perceptions of Life Quality*, with kind permission from Plenum Publishing Corporation, NY.

Table 3.1 Noack, (1991), in Badura and Kickbusch, *Health Promotion Research: Towards a New Social Epidemiology*, reproduced with kind permission from World Health Organisation European Regional Publications, Copenhagen.

Table 3.2, Perinatal and Infant Mortality in Europe. Crown copyright, reproduced with permission of the Controller of Her Majesty's Stationery Office.

Table 3.4, from *U205 Book 3 The Health of Nations*, (1985), reproduced with kind permission of The Open University Press, Milton Keynes.

Figure 4.1, The Development of Health Promotion from Bunton & McDonald, (1992), *Health Promotion, Discipline and Diversity*, reproduced with permission from Routledge, London.

Figures 12.3, 5.1, 5.3, 5.4, from the *Health Education Journal* reproduced with permission of the Health Education Authority.
Table 12.1, from Killoran, (1992), *Putting Health into Contracts*, reproduced by kind permission of the Health Education Authority.
Figure 13.4 Superman poster.
Pregnant man poster Chapter 4, © Saatchi and Saatchi, reproduced with their permission.
All by kind permission of the Health Education Authority.

Figure 6.1, The Ethical Grid, from Seedhouse, D, (1988), in *Ethics, The Heart of Health Care*, p.141, reproduced with permission from John Wiley & Sons Ltd, Chichester, UK.

Figure 6.2, Andy Capp cartoon used in the Health Education Authority's *Look After Your Heart* campaign. Reproduced with permission from Mirror Group Newspapers. Distributed by North America Syndicate.

Figure 10.2, 'Heroin really screws you up poster.' Crown copyright, reproduced with the permission of the Controller of Her Majesty's Stationery Office.

Figure 10.3, The Theory of Reasoned Action (from Azjen and Fishbein), in: Understanding Attitudes and Predicting Social Behaviour, Azjen and Fishbein (Eds), © 1990, pp. 5–11. Reprinted by permission of Prentice-Hall, Inc., Englewood Cliffs, N.J.

Figure 12.1, Rational Health Planning, McCarthy, (1982), From *Epidemiology and Policies for Health Planning*, reproduced with kind permission of the King's Fund Centre.

Figure 12.4, from Ewles and Simnett, (1992), *Promoting Health: A Practical Guide to Health Education*, reproduced by kind permission of Scutari Press, London.

Figure 12.5, from Green *et al.*, (1980), *Health Education Planning: A Diagnostic Approach*, by kind permission of Mayfield Publishing Co., Mountain View, CA.

Figure 12.6, A Systems Approach to Health Education Planning, (1986); Figure 10.3, Education for Health diagram, (1990); Figure 7.2, The Model of Radical Health Promotion, reproduced with permission from Professor Keith Tones, Director, Health Education Unit, Leeds Metropolitan University, UK.

Author's Acknowledgements

We wish to acknowledge the contribution colleagues and students at the University of the West of England and South Bank University have made to this book. Their experience, ideas and commitment to furthering the practice of health promotion prompted us to write this book. They are too numerous to name, but thanks especially to Judy Orme and Tricia Parsons. We do of course take full responsibility for any inaccuracies and errors.

Finally we would like to thank our families and partners for their support and patience. A special debt of gratitude is owed to Stephen Wills who was unfailingly encouraging during the writing of this book but sadly he died before its publication.

Introduction

Health promotion is an important part of the work of a wide range of health care workers, and those engaged in education and social welfare. It is an emerging area of practice and study, still defining its boundaries. This book is intended to provide a theoretical framework which is vital if health promoters are to be clear about their intentions and desired outcomes when they embark on interventions designed to promote health. It offers a foundation for practice which encourages practitioners to see the potential for health promotion in their work.

The book is divided into three main sections. The first section provides a theoretical background, exploring the concepts of health, health education and health promotion. It concludes that health promotion is the working towards positive health and well-being of individuals, groups and communities. Health promotion includes health education but also acknowledges that it is social and economic factors which determine health status. Those who promote health thus need to be clear about their intentions and how they perceive the purpose of health promotion. Is it, for example, to encourage healthy lifestyles? Or is it to redress health inequalities and empower people to take more control over their lives? We shall be asking readers to reflect on these and other questions in the context of their own work.

The second section discusses some of the practice issues for the health promoter, in particular the ethical and political dilemmas that face a reflective practitioner. Two strategies which are especially problematic are selected for further investigation – community development and behaviour change. How can health promoters work with communities and what are the strengths and limitations of a community development approach? What influences individual health behaviour and how can we help people to change? We also outline the main agencies that practise health promotion and in view of recommendations in the 'Health of the Nation' strategy to set up 'healthy alliances', we consider how individuals and organizations can work together.

Section 3 is concerned with the implementation of health promotion. How do we assess clients' needs? Should health promotion interventions be targeted to particular groups? What strategies have been successful and what needs to be taken into account when planning an intervention or health promotion programme? Above all, how will we know if health promotion works?

This book is suitable for a wide range of professional groups and the examples and case studies have been chosen to reflect the diversity of people who practise health promotion. It includes many interactive exercises to encourage reflection and debate and to enable the reader to apply their knowledge and increased understanding to practice situations. Where appropriate, feedback has been given but on many occasions this is not possible because the issues are open ended and contested. The important aim though, is to acknowledge that readers will have to consider these issues for themselves, and not have their views prescribed or limited.

The book is clearly structured and signposted for ease of reading and study. Each chapter starts with an overview outlining the contents of that chapter and its links with other chapters and a few key points. A chapter summary acts as an *aide-mémoire* of the main points covered. Interspersed throughout the text are a number of helpful **Example**, **Activity** and **Discussion** boxes:

☞ = content input as an **Example**;

? = **Activity**, in general more linked to text and some responses discussed;

✦ = **Discussion** point, broader and more open ended.

Each chapter includes recommendations for further reading, and questions to encourage further discussion and debate either by the individual reader or student groups. We hope that this book will encourage readers to develop their practice and thus contribute to the challenge of promoting people's health.

An aid for the reflective practitioner, this book will help the student in basic or post-basic training and the qualified professional who wants to include health promotion in their work.

SECTION 1
The Theory of Health Promotion

This section explores the concepts of health, health education and health promotion. Those who promote health need to be clear about their intentions and how they perceive the purpose of health promotion. Is it to encourage healthy lifestyles? Or is it to redress health inequalities and empower people to take control over their lives?

1 Concepts of health
2 Influences on health
3 Measuring health
4 The development of health education
   and health promotion
5 Models and approaches to health
   promotion

Concepts of health 1

Overview

Everyone engaged in the task of promoting health starts with a view of what health is. However, there is a wide variety of these views, or concepts, of health. It is important at the outset to be clear about the concepts of health which you personally adhere to, and to recognize where these differ from those of your colleagues and clients. Otherwise, you may find yourself drawn into conflicts about appropriate strategies and advice that are actually due to different ideas concerning the end goal of health. This chapter introduces different concepts of health, and traces the origin of these views. Working your way through this chapter will enable you to clarify your own views on the definition of health and to locate these views in a conceptual framework.

Key points
■ Disease
■ Illness
■ Ill health
■ Health as:
  ■ Holistic
  ■ The product of
    Western scientific
    medicine
  ■ Socially
    constructed
  ■ Autonomy
■ Lay health beliefs
■ Cultural health
  beliefs

Defining health, disease, illness and ill health

Health

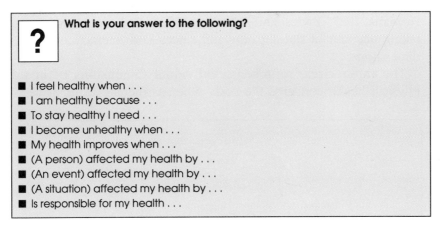

? What is your answer to the following?

■ I feel healthy when . . .
■ I am healthy because . . .
■ To stay healthy I need . . .
■ I become unhealthy when . . .
■ My health improves when . . .
■ (A person) affected my health by . . .
■ (An event) affected my health by . . .
■ (A situation) affected my health by . . .
■ Is responsible for my health . . .

Health is a broad concept which can embody a huge range of meanings, from the narrowly technical to the all-embracing moral or philosophical. The word "health" is derived from whole, hale and healing, signalling that health concerns the whole person and his or her integrity, soundness, or well-being. There are "common sense" views of health which are passed through generations as part of a common cultural heritage. These are termed "lay" concepts of health, and everyone acquires a knowledge of this through their socialization into society. Different societies or different groups within one society have different views on what constitutes "common sense".

Health has two common meanings in everyday use, one negative and one positive. The negative definition of health is the absence of disease or illness. This is the meaning of health within the Western scientific medical model, which is explored in greater detail later on in this chapter. The positive definition of health is a state of well-being. "Health is a state of complete physical, mental and social well-being, not merely the absence of disease or infirmity" (World Health Organisation, 1946).

> **?** **Which definitions are being used in the following extract?**
>
> Jane left for school feeling normal and able to perform her best in class. By break-time, she was feeling hot and sweaty. She told her teacher she felt shaky, and asked to be excused from outside play. Her teacher sent her to the school nurse, who took her temperature with a thermometer. The thermometer reading was 101 degrees. The school nurse rang her mother and told her Jane had complained of feeling unwell, and that she was running a temperature. Jane was sent home and stayed off school for two days.

Some authors argue that health is holistic and includes different dimensions which each need to be considered (Aggleton and Homans 1987; Ewles and Simnett, 1992). Holistic health means taking account of the separate influences and interaction of these dimensions.

The inner circle represents individual dimensions of health. Physical health concerns the body whereas mental health concerns

Figure 1.1 Dimensions of health. Adapted from Aggleton and Homans (1987) and Ewles and Simnett (1992).

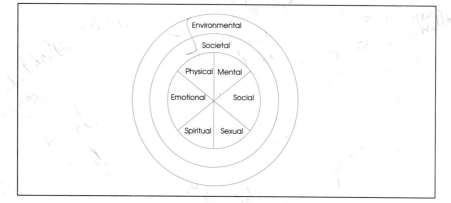

the ability to think and make judgements. Emotional health refers to the recognition and appropriate discharge of feeling states. Social health concerns the integration of somebody in a web of social relationships. Spritual health is the recognition and ability to put into practice moral or religious principles or beliefs. Sexual health is the acceptance and ability to achieve a satisfactory expression of one's sexuality.

The two outer circles are broader dimensions of health which affect the individual. Societal health refers to the link between health and the way a society is structured. This includes the basic infrastructure necessary for health (for example, shelter, peace, food, income), and the degree of integration or division within society. "Health can only be shared. There is no health for me without my brother. There is no health for Britain without Bangladesh" (Wilson, 1975). We shall see in Chapter 2 how the existence of patterned inequalities between groups of people harms health. Environmental health refers to the physical environment in which people live, and includes things such as housing, transport, sanitation and pure water facilities and pollution.

From your own experience identify one positive and one negative example of health from each of the dimensions of health.

Disease, illness and ill health

Disease, illness and ill health are often used interchangeably. Disease is the objective state of ill health, which may be verified by accepted canons of proof. In our society, these accepted canons of proof are couched in the language of scientific medicine. For example, microscopic analysis may yield evidence of changes in cell structure, which may in turn lead to a diagnosis of cancer or disease. Disease is the existence of some pathology or abnormality of the body which is capable of detection.

Illness is the subjective experience of loss of health. This is couched in terms of symptoms, for example, the reporting of aches or pains, or loss of function. Illness and disease are not the same, although there is a large degree of co-existence. For example, someone may be diagnosed as having cancer through screening even when there have been no reported symptoms. That is, someone may be diagnosed as having a disease although they have not reported any illness. When someone reports symptoms, and further investigations such as blood tests prove a disease process, the two concepts, disease and illness, coincide. In these instances, the term ill health is used. Ill health is therefore an umbrella term used to refer to the experience of disease plus illness.

Some people, such as doctors and nurses, acquire a specialized view of health. This specialist view is gained through their professional training. During professional training health workers are introduced to their field of knowledge, and they spend much of their time with other students and practitioners. They learn to use professional jargon, and adopt the meanings and value systems of their peers. This process is called secondary socialization.

In modern Western societies, and in many other societies as well, the dominant professional view of health adopted by most health care workers during their training and practice is labelled Western scientific medicine. Western scientific medicine operates with a narrow view of health, which is often used to refer to no disease or no illness. In this sense, health is a negative term, defined more by what it is not than by what it is.

These definitions become powerful because they are used by professionals, and because they are used in a variety of contexts, not just in professional circles. For example, the media often presents this view of health, disease and illness, in dramas set in hospitals or in documentaries about health issues. By these means, professional definitions become known and accepted in society at large.

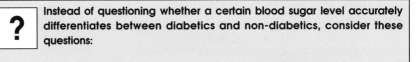

? Instead of questioning whether a certain blood sugar level accurately differentiates between diabetics and non-diabetics, consider these questions:

- Why is it important to make this distinction?
- Who stands to gain from such a process?
- Whose livelihood depends on the business of investigation, diagnosis, and treatment?
- How does the person receiving a diagnosis of diabetes experience the process?
- Why don't all diabetics comply with a prescribed treatment regime?

The Western scientific medical model of health

This view of health is extremely influential, as it underpins much of the training and ethos of a wide variety of health workers. The scientific medical model arose in Western Europe at the time of the Enlightenment, with the rise of rationality and science as forms of knowledge. In earlier times, religion provided a way of knowing and understanding the world.

The Enlightenment changed the old order, and substituted science for religion as the dominant means of knowledge and understanding. This was accompanied by a proliferation of equipment and techniques for studying the world. The invention of the microscope and telescope revealed whole worlds which before had been invisible. Observation, calculation and classification became the means of increasing knowledge. Such knowledge was put to practical purposes, and applied science was one of the forces which accompanied the Industrial Revolution. In an atmosphere when everything was deemed knowable through the proper application of scientific method, the human body became a key object for the pursuit of scientific knowledge. What could be seen, and measured, and catalogued, was "true" in an objective and universal sense.

☞ **Key milestones in the development of scientific medicine.**

1543 Vesalius publishes *On the Structure of the Human Body* based on his own dissections
1628 Harvey publishes his discoveries concerning the blood circulatory system
1674 Leeuwenhoek produces lenses powerful enough to enable him to observe bacteria
1796 Jenner first uses vaccine derived from cowpox to successfully immunize a person against smallpox
1858 Virchow publishes a book on cellular pathology which introduces the concept of the cell as the centre of all pathological changes
1864 Pasteur isolates organisms under the microscope
1865 Lister begins the practice of antisepsis during surgery, which is followed by a dramatic reduction in mortality rates
1882 Koch isolates the tubercle bacillus
1883 Koch isolates the cholera bacillus
1895 Roentgen discovers X-rays
1900 Landsteiner discovers the four human blood types A, B, AB and O

This view of health is characterized as:

■ **Biomedical** – health is assumed to be a property of biological beings.
■ **Reductionist** – states of being such as health and disease may be reduced to smaller and smaller constitutive components of the biological body.
■ **Mechanistic** – it conceptualizes and treats the body as if it was a machine.
■ **Allopathic** – it works by a system of opposites. If something is wrong with a body, treatment consists of applying an opposite force to correct the sickness, e.g. pharmacological drugs which combat the sickness.

Doyal and Doyal (1984) develop the machine analogy further, and refer to five basic assumptions underpinning Western scientific medicine. These are:

1. The body is like a machine, in which all the parts are interconnected but capable of being separated and treated separately.

2. Health equals all the parts of the body functioning properly.
3. Illness equals some malfunction of the parts of the body, which is measurable.
4. Disease is caused by internal processes such as degeneration through ageing or the failure of self-regulation, or by external processes such as the invasion of pathogens into the body.
5. Medical treatment aims to restore normal functioning or health to the body system.

This view equates health with "normality". This also conveys a notion of morality, thus "normal equals good".

? **The causes of infertility are thought to be shared equally between men and women.**

Negative terms are used in medical textbooks to refer to the female reproductive system:
■ Incompetent cervix
■ Blighted ovum
■ Blocked fallopian tubes
■ Irregular menstrual cycles
■ Imbalances of the hormone system
■ Hostile cervical mucus.
The male reproductive system is referred to in positive terms:
■ Vigorous or motile sperm
■ Robust
■ Morphologically sound (Pfeffer, 1985).
Can you think of other examples of medical discourse that reflect a moral value?

New developments in medicine and nursing recognize the importance of social factors in the causation of health and disease, and the necessity of treating the whole person. Nowadays, sociology and social policy are included as part of the curriculum for nurses and other health workers. However, the legacy of Western scientific medicine is pervasive, and elements of this approach still underpin the professional training of many health workers.

"There is a dichotomy between therapeutic medicine and preventive medicine which exists both at community level and clinical level. One of the main reasons for the dichotomy must be the traditional undergraduate and postgraduate training which produces doctors who are largely unaware of the potential for prevention of chronic disease but who have an exaggerated view of the benefits of treatment" (National Forum for CHD Prevention, 1990, p.46).

A critique of scientific medicine

The role of medicine in determining health

The view that health is the absence of disease and illness, and that medical treatment can restore the body to good health has been criticized. The distribution of health and ill health has been analysed from a historical and social science perspective. It has been argued that medicine is not as effective as is often claimed. The 20th century has seen a steady reduction in mortality and increased longevity amongst people living in the industrialized West, and it is often assumed that medical advances have been responsible for this. McKeown and Lowe (1974) set out to test this assumption by undertaking a historical analysis (see Figure 1.2 on page 10).

? **What effect do medical advances in knowledge have on death rates? What other reasons could account for declining death rates?**

McKeown and Lowe (1974) concluded that social advances in general living conditions, such as improved sanitation and nutrition, have been responsible for most of the reduction in mortality achieved during the last century. The contribution of medicine to reduced mortality has been minor, when compared with the major impact of improved environmental conditions.

Cochrane (1972) argues that most medical interventions have not been proved effective prior to their widespread adoption. The randomized controlled trial is the scientific method of validating a medical treatment as effective. This method relies on randomly dividing people with the same disease or illness into two groups. One group receives the medical treatment, whilst the other group does not. The two groups are then compared, and only when the group receiving medical treatment fares significantly better is the treatment deemed effective. Cochrane (1972) argues that it is relatively rare for experimental treatments to be properly evaluated using randomized controlled trials. Often the demand for treatment or a cure makes such trials impossible. A recent example of this is the demand by people with AIDS to receive the new drug AZT whilst it is still at the experimental stage. Medical treatments may be adopted even when they have not been shown to be effective. For example, coronary care units have grown in number, although there is no evidence that hospital care produces better outcomes than home care (Skrabanek and McCormick, 1992).

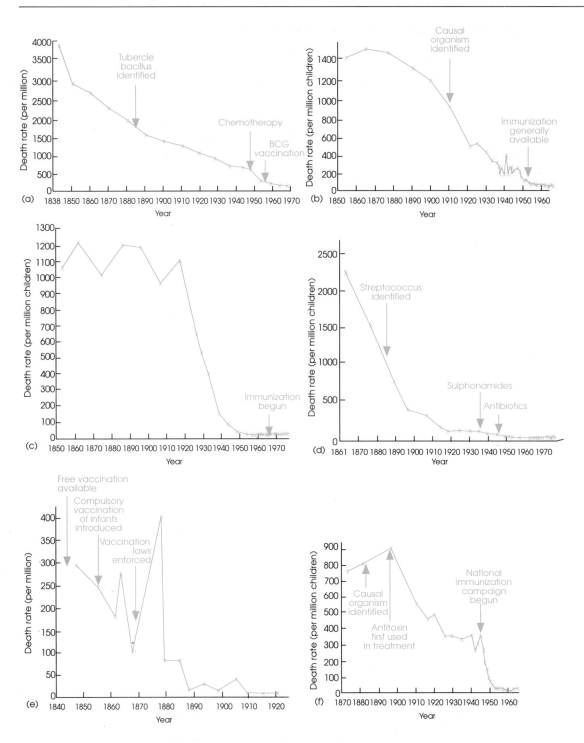

Figure 1.2 The role of medicine in reducing mortality.

(a) Respiratory tuberculosis, England and Wales.

(b) Whooping cough; death rates of children under 15, England and Wales.

(c) Measles: death rates of children under 15, England and Wales.

(d) Scarlet fever: death rates of children under 15, England and Wales.

(e) Small pox: death rates, England and Wales.

(f) Diphtheria: death rates of children under 15, England and Wales. From McKeown and Lowe (1974).

The role of social factors in determining health

The fact that inequalities in health between different social classes have not been reduced, but have actually increased since the post World War Two boom, gives further credence to the importance of social factors in determining health (Townsend *et al.*, 1988). As Chapter 2 will show, the distribution of health mirrors the distribution of material resources within society. In general, the more equal a society is in its distribution of resources, the more equal, and better, is the health status of its citizens (Open University, 1985; Wilkinson, 1992). Modern Britain is characterized by profound inequalities in income and wealth (Rose, 1993). These in turn are associated with persistent inequalities in health (Townsend *et al.*, 1988). The impact of scientific medicine on health is marginal when compared to major structural features such as the distribution of wealth, income, housing and employment.

Social scientists have provided a critique of scientific medicine by going beyond its frame of reference and challenging medicine's claims to objective truth. The two main claims of social scientists are that health and illness are social constructs, and that medicine is a social activity.

Health as a social construct

Social scientists view health and disease as socially constructed entities. Health and disease are not states of objective reality waiting to be uncovered and investigated by scientific medicine. Rather, they are actively produced and negotiated by ordinary people. This process becomes most apparent when doctors and their patients disagree about the significance or meaning of symptoms. For example, someone can feel ill but after investigations nothing medically wrong can be found. The subjective experience of feeling ill is not always matched by an objective diagnosis of disease. When this happens, doctors and health workers may label such sufferers "malingerers", denying the validity of subjective illness. This can have important consequences, for example a sick certificate may be withheld if a doctor is not convinced that someone's reported illness is genuine.

In November 1993 Judge John Prosser, Q.C. decided that RSI (repetitive strain injury, a work related condition) does not exist and dismissed a claim for compensation. Judge Prosser said RSI is "meaningless" and "has no place in the medical books". He described RSI sufferers as "eggshell personalities who need to get a grip on themselves".

Can you think of other examples of a disease or condition which has been experienced by people but not been readily diagnosed?

Do you know anybody who has experienced symptoms without being given a diagnosis?

Figure 1.3 The relationship between disease and illness.

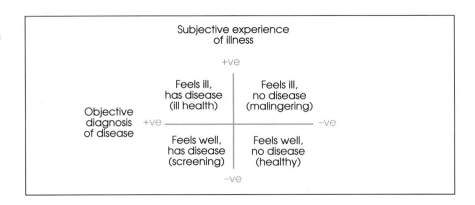

It is also possible to experience no symptoms or signs of disease, but to be labelled sick as a result of examination or screening. Hypertension and precancerous changes to cell structures are two examples where screening may identify a disease even though the person concerned feels perfectly healthy. Figure 1.3 gives a visual representation of these discrepancies. The central point is that subjective perceptions cannot be overruled, or invalidated, by scientific medicine.

Medicine as a means of social control

Social scientists argue that medicine is a social enterprise closely linked with the exercise of professional power (Stacey, 1988). Medicine, it is argued, is not a value-free activity, undertaken altruistically by benefactors. Rather, it is a powerful means of social control, whereby the categories of disease, illness, madness and deviancy are used to maintain a *status quo* in society.

The following is a list of labels which are attached to people at certain stages of their life. Some are universal (everyone is born and dies), others only happen to some people at some stages of their lives. For each label identify:

■ Who is responsible for attaching the label in a recognized, or socially approved, manner, as part of their professional duties?
■ Who is likely to receive the label?
■ What are the likely consequences of being so labelled?
  ■ Birth
  ■ Death
  ■ Illness requiring a prescription
  ■ Illness requiring a sick certificate
  ■ Long-term or chronic illness
  ■ Being in need of continual care and attendance
  ■ Being disabled
  ■ Mental illness
  ■ Mental illness requiring hospitalization
  ■ Having a child on the at risk register
  ■ Having a learning difficulty

> **(cont.)**
> ■ Being convicted of a crime
> ■ Terminal illness requiring hospice care.

Doctors who make the diagnosis are in a powerful position. Access to such power is controlled by professional associations with their own vested interests to protect (Freidson, 1986). The 1858 Medical Act established the General Medical Council which was authorized to regulate doctors, oversee medical education, and keep a register of qualified practitioners. Medical colleges resisted the entry of women to the profession for many years (Stacey, 1988). In 1901 there were 36 000 medical practitioners, of whom 212 were women. There is evidence that Black and Asian doctors face discrimination in their medical careers (Skellington and Morris, 1992; Esmail and Everington, 1993). This implies that ability is not the sole criterion for gaining a place to train in medicine or in subsequent career progression. Medicine may be seen as a social activity which concentrates professional power amongst an elite.

A stronger form of this argument says that medicine upholds a specific form of economy (capitalism), and/or patriarchy (the institutionalized power of men over women). For a capitalist state to thrive, social order and healthy workers are needed, and the National Health Service (NHS) provides the means to achieve both (Doyal with Pennell, 1979). Some feminists argue that the NHS primarily serves the needs of men, and that women's health needs tend to be subordinated to their role as mother, wife and carer. These issues are discussed in greater detail in Chapter 2.

Health as autonomy

It has been claimed that health means autonomy and that autonomy or health is subverted by the medicalization of life (Illich, 1975). This critique argues that medicine has acquired an authority beyond its legitimate area of operation. The medicalization of life is the encroachment of medical decisions and techniques into ordinary stages of the life cycle, such as birth and death. Doctors are called upon to make life and death decisions; yet they have no particular training which qualifies them to make these moral choices. Illich argues that this kind of power does not naturally belong to technical experts but is a fundamental human right which should be exercised by everyone in relation to their own lives, if they are to be healthy.

For Illich, health is a personal task which people must be free to pursue autonomously. Doctors and health workers contribute to ill health by taking over people's responsibility for their health. In addition, the practice of medicine leads to iatrogenic ill health caused by doctors and health workers. Illich identifies three types of iatrogenesis. Clinical iatrogenesis is ill health caused by medical intervention, for example, side-effects caused by prescribed medicine, dependency on prescribed drugs and cross-infection in medical settings such as hospitals. Social iatrogenesis is the loss of coping and the right to self-care which has resulted from the medicalization of everyday life. Cultural iatrogenesis is the loss of the means whereby people cope with pain and suffering, which results from the unrealistic expectations generated by medicine.

Health workers come to be seen as disabling elements in the lives of ordinary people. Whilst it is possible to agree with Illich that doctors and health workers wield enormous power in people's lives, which is not always exercised in accordance with their patients' wishes or beliefs, it does not follow that we would all be better off without any health care system at all. Medicine has made some remarkable inroads on people's health (for example, the widespread use of antibiotics in the 1950s). The caring function of health workers is also important for many people when they are ill, especially for those without close ties of family and friends. To argue, as Illich does, for the abolition of professional health workers seems to be a case of throwing the baby out with the bath water.

The view that people should make their own decisions about their own health and that of their dependants is widespread amongst both the general public and government circles. The rise of self-help groups dating from the 1970s is an example of how popular this view is (Lock, 1986). The huge increase in the number of people involved in self-help health activities indicates a general belief that people know what's best for them, and that other people in similar circumstances are often more helpful and supportive than medical experts. This view is mirrored in official policy documents. The Government's recent pronouncements on the importance of "consumerism" in health service delivery reinforces the belief that self-determination and autonomy are intrinsic to health: ". . . the purpose of all the reforms in this White Paper is to provide a better service for patients . . ." (Department of Health, 1989, p.6). This includes shorter waiting times, better waiting room facilities, more information about treatment, rapid notification of results of medical tests, clear complaints procedures, and "a wider range of optional extras and amenities for patients who want to pay for them – such as single rooms, personal telephones, televisions, and a wider choice of meals" (Department of Health, 1989, p.7)

Lay concepts of health

For people concerned with the promotion of health, there is another problem with the dominance of scientific medicine. This is the focus within medicine on illness and disease, and the neglect of health as a positive concept in its own right. Many researchers have studied the general public's beliefs about health or lay concepts of health. The findings present an interesting picture, where there are continuities in definitions but also differences attributable to age, sex and class.

Herzlich (1973) studied a group of middle-class Parisians and Normans, and found they described health in three different ways:

- As a state of being and the absence of illness
- As something to have, an inner strength or resistance to ill health
- As a state of doing and being able to fulfil the maximum potential for life.

Williams (1983) studied a group of older people from Aberdeen who defined health as wholeness or integrity, inner strength and ability to cope. People suffering from disease could be described as healthy if they met these criteria.

 "Health is not a state of being . . . it is a process of adaptation to the changing demands of living and the changing meanings we give to life" (Dubos, 1960).

Other researchers have identified a social class difference in concepts of health (d'Houtaud and Field, 1986; Calnan, 1987; Blaxter, 1990). Middle-class respondents typically have a more positive view of health, as something which is linked to enjoying life, and being fit and active. Working-class respondents tend to see health as more functional, to do with getting through the day and not being ill.

Functional health means being able to do those normal social tasks which are expected of someone and is: "the state of optimum capacity of an individual for the effective performance of the roles and tasks for which (s)he has been socialised" (Parsons, 1972, p.117). Blaxter (1990) identifies a gender difference, with men having a more positive notion of health as being fit, and women having a more negative notion of health as not being ill and being able to carry out everyday tasks.

One way of thinking about these differences is in terms of internal and external locus of control. These terms are used in psychology to refer to people's beliefs about how much choice and self-determination they have, and are explored in more detail in

Chapter 10. A person with a strong internal locus of control believes they have the power to make decisions which will affect their life. They will therefore be strongly motivated to make recommended changes to improve their health. By contrast, the person with a strong external locus of control believes they are relatively powerless to make changes which will affect their life. They are more likely to be fatalistic about the future and will not be strongly motivated to make recommended changes to improve their health.

Researchers have found that these differing views are linked to social class. Typically, middle class people are more likely to have a strong internal locus of control. Working-class people are more likely to have a strong external locus of control.

> **?** What explanations can you think of to account for this finding?

Part of the explanation might be that, compared to working class people, middle class people have more control over their lives due to higher income, better housing and more job security. This in turn can lead to different social classes holding different beliefs about autonomy or fatalism, which are then passed on to children.

Official and lay health beliefs

There is then a difference between lay and professional concepts of health. The gap between the two has been identified by health workers as a problem, giving rise to concern. The concern centres around two issues, the perceived lack of communication or poor communication between health worker and client, and clients' lack of compliance with prescribed treatment regimes. However, there is a crossover between lay and professional beliefs about health.

Health workers acquire their professional view of health during training. These beliefs overlay their original views of health adopted at an early age from family and society, so professionals are familiar with both. The general public is also aware of, and operates with, both sets of beliefs. So the two sets of beliefs, scientific medicine and lay public, are not discrete entities but overlap each other and exist in tandem.

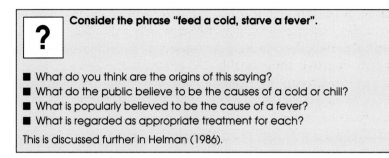

? Consider the phrase "feed a cold, starve a fever".

■ What do you think are the origins of this saying?
■ What do the public believe to be the causes of a cold or chill?
■ What is popularly believed to be the cause of a fever?
■ What is regarded as appropriate treatment for each?

This is discussed further in Helman (1986).

Cornwell (1984) describes how people operate with both offical and lay beliefs about health. Cornwell's study of London's Eastenders found that accounts of health were either public or private. Public accounts are couched in terms of scientific medicine and reflect these dominant beliefs. Health and illness are related to medical diagnosis and treatment, and medical terms and events are used to explain health status. These public accounts were offered first in Cornwell's interviews. What Cornwell terms private accounts reflect lay views of health, which typically use more holistic and social concepts to explain health and illness. For example, private accounts relate health to general life experiences, such as employment, housing and perceived stress. Private accounts were offered in subsequent interviews, when a relationship had been established between Cornwell and the women she was interviewing. Cornwell suggests that people are therefore aware of both systems of beliefs and can use either when asked to talk about health. In encounters with strangers who are perceived as professionals, people use public accounts. However, in more informal settings, people use private accounts.

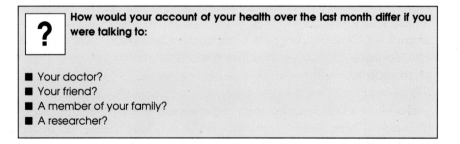

? How would your account of your health over the last month differ if you were talking to:

■ Your doctor?
■ Your friend?
■ A member of your family?
■ A researcher?

Cultural views of health

We are able to think about health using the language of scientific medicine because that is part of our cultural heritage. We do so as a matter of course, and think it is self-evident or commonsense. However, other societies and cultures have their own common-sense ways of talking about health which are very different. The Ashanti view disease as the outcome of malign human or supernatural agencies, and diagnosis is a matter of determining who has been offended. Treatment includes ceremonies to propitiate these spirits as an integral part of the process. Ways of thinking about health and disease reflect the basic preoccupations of society, and dominant views of society and the world. Anthropologists refer to this phenomenon as the cultural specificity of notions of health and disease.

 The Gnau of New Guinea refer to illness and other general misfortunes by the same word, *wola*. They also use the pidgin English *sik* to refer to bodily misfortunes. Sickness is a particular type of misfortune which is caused by evil beings or by magic and sorcery. People who are sick act in certain ways (shunning certain foods, eating alone) which oblige others to find out and treat the illness.
Source: Lewis, 1986.

In any multicultural society such as Britain, a variety of cultural views co-exist at any one time. For example, traditional Chinese medicine is based on the dichotomy of Ying and Yang, female and male, hot and cold, which is applied to symptoms, diet and treatments, such as acupuncture and Chinese herbal medicine. Alternative practitioners offer therapies based on these cultural views of health and disease alongside (or increasingly within) the National Health Service, which is based on scientific medicine.

The influence of culture on views of health is most apparent when other societies are being studied. However, Crawford (1984) applies the same analysis to Western society, with provocative results. Crawford argues that capitalism is the bedrock of Western society. Capitalism is an economic system centred on maximum production and consumption of goods through the free market. These economic goals have their parallel in views about health. Health is concerned with both release (consumption) and discipline (production). Hence the co-existence of apparently opposite beliefs in relation to health.

Figure 1.4 Cultural views about health in capitalist society. Adapted from Crawford (1984).

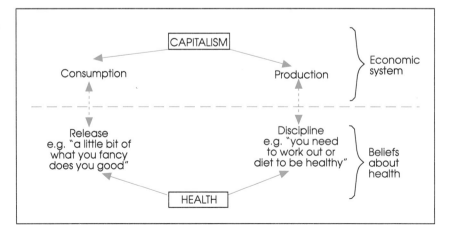

A unified view of health

Is there any unifying concept of health which can reconcile these different views and beliefs? Attempts at such a synthesis have come from philosophers such as Seedhouse (1986) and from organizations concerned with health such as the World Health Organisation. Seedhouse attempts a grand synthesis of different theories of health from a philosophical perspective. Figure 1.5 gives a diagrammatic representation of this.

? | **Seedhouse identifies four theories of health.**
What problems can you identify with each of these four views of health?

"Health as an ideal state" provides a holistic and positive definition of health. However, it has been argued that this definition is too idealistic and vague to provide practical guidance for health promoters. Health in this sense is probably unattainable.

The functional view of health imposes social norms without regard to individual variation. It ignores the fact that these social norms (for example, homophobia or sexism) may themselves be contributing to ill health. It also excludes people who, due to a chronic illness or disability, are unable to fulfil normal social roles, such as employees. Using a functional definition of health, a contented and coping person who has a disability can never be counted as healthy.

The view of health as a commodity leads to unrealistic expectations. Health cannot be guaranteed by paying a higher price for health care. This view also compartmentalizes the total experience of health or ill health into different sections. This is at odds with how people experience health and illness.

Health as autonomy and integrity focuses on individual circumstances and the ability to cope with change, but does not address the social environment which creates health and ill health.

Seedhouse suggests that these four views can be combined in a unified theory of health as the foundations for achievement. This definition includes the notion of autonomy as crucial to health and acknowledges that people have different starting points which set limits for their potential for health. It encompasses a positive notion of health which is applicable to everyone, whatever their circumstances. However, it could be argued that this definition does not acknowledge the social construction of health sufficiently. People as individuals have little scope to determine optimum conditions for realizing their potential.

The theory that health is an ideal state:

■ A "Socratic" goal of perfect well-being in every respect.

■ An end in itself.

■ Disease, illness, handicap, and social problems must be absent.

A group of theories which hold that health is a personal strength or ability – either physical, metaphysical or intellectual:

■ These strengths and abilities are not commodities which can be given or purchased. Nor are they ideal states. They are developed as personal tasks. They can be lost. They can be encouraged.

The theory that health is the foundations for achievement of potentials

"A person's optimum state of health is equivalent to the state of the set of conditions which fulfil or enable a person to work to fulfil his or her realistic chosen and biological potentials. Some of these conditions are of highest importance for all people. Others are variable dependent upon individual abilities and circumstances." (p. 61)

– Created by removing obstacles

The theory that health is a commodity which can be bought or given:

■ The rationale which lies behind medical theory and practice.

■ Usually an end for the provider, a means for the receiver.

■ Health is lost in the presence of disease, illness, pain, malady. It might be restored piecemeal.

The theory that health is the physical and mental fitness to do socialized daily tasks (i.e., to function normally in a person's own society):

■ A means towards the end of normal social functioning.

■ All disabling disease, illness and handicap must be absent.

Figure 1.5 A summary of theories of health. Adapted from Seedhouse (1986).

"By health I mean the power to live a full, adult, living, breathing life in close contact with what I love . . . I want to be all that I am capable of becoming" (Mansfield, 1977, p.278).

The view of health as personal potential is attractive because it is so flexible, but this very flexibility causes problems. It leads to relativism (health may mean a thousand different things to a thousand different people), which makes it impracticable as a working definition for health promoters.

The World Health Organisation (WHO) has been responsible for progressing the debate about definitions of health.

"[Health is] the extent to which an individual or group is able, on the one hand, to realise aspirations and satisfy needs; and, on the other hand, to change or cope with the environment. Health is, therefore, seen as a resource for everyday life, not an object of living; it is a positive concept emphasising social and personal resources, as well as physical capacities" (WHO, 1984).

This definition is important for several reasons. It establishes health as a social as well as an individual product, and it emphasizes the dynamic and positive nature of health. Health is viewed as both a fundamental human right and a sound social investment. It provides a variety of reasons for supporting health, which are likely to meet the concerns of a range of groups. This definition of health establishes a broad consensus for prioritizing health, and legitimizes a range of activities designed to promote health. For example, in addition to the more acceptable strategies of primary health care and personal skills development, the WHO has also identified the more radical strategies of community participation and healthy public policy as essential to the promotion of health (WHO, 1986). However, it could still be argued that such a broad definition makes it difficult to identify practical priorities for health promotion activities.

There is no agreement on what is meant by health. Health is used in many different contexts to refer to many different aspects of life. Given this complexity of meanings, it is unlikely that a unified concept of health which includes all its meanings will be formulated.

Conclusion

There are no rights and wrongs regarding concepts of health. Different people are likely to hold different views of health and may operate with several conflicting views simultaneously. Where people are located socially, in terms of social class, gender, ethnic origin and occupation, will affect their concept of health. There is such a range of meaning attached to the notion of health, that in any particular situation, it is important to find out what views are in operation. Clarifying what you understand by health, and what other people mean when they talk about health, is an essential first step for the health promoter.

Questions for further discussion

■ How would you describe your own concept of health?
■ What have been the most important influences on your views?

Summary

Definitions of health arise from many different perspectives. Whilst scientific medicine is the most powerful ideology in the West, it is not all-embracing. Social sciences' perspectives on health produce a powerful critique of scientific medicine, and point to the importance of social factors in the construction and meaning of health. Lay concepts of health derived from different cultures co-exist alongside scientific medicine. Attempts to produce a unified concept of health appear to founder through over-generalization and vagueness.

Further reading

Aggleton P (1990) *Health*, London, Routledge.

A readable introduction to a social science perspective on health.

Seedhouse D (1986) *Health: The Foundations for Achievement. John Wiley & Sons.*

A clear account of different views of health which attempts to provide a unified concept of health.

Currer C and Stacey M (eds) *Concepts of Health, Illness and Disease: A Comparative Perspective*, Leamington Spa, Berg.

An edited selection of research into different cultural concepts of health.

References

Aggleton P (1990) *Health*, London, Routledge.

Aggleton P and Homans H (1987) *Educating about AIDS*, NHS Training Authority.

Blaxter M (1990) *Health and Lifestyles*, London, Tavistock/ Routledge.

Calnan M (1987) *Health and Illness*, London, Tavistock.

Cochrane AL (1972) *Effectiveness and Efficiency*, The Nuffield Provincial Hospitals Trust.

Cornwell J (1984) *Hard-earned Lives*, London, Tavistock.

Crawford R (1984) "A cultural account of 'health': control, release and the social body", in McKinley J (ed.) *Issues in the Political Economy of Health Care*, pp. 60–103 London, Tavistock.

Department of Health (1989) *Working for Patients*, London, HMSO.

Doyal L and Doyal L (1984) in Birke L and Silvertown J (eds.) *More than the Parts: Biology and Politics*, London, Pluto Press.

Doyal L with Pennell I (1979) *The Political Economy of Health*, London, Pluto Press.

Dubos R (1960) *Mirage of health*, London, Allen and Unwin.

Esmail A and Everington S (1993) "Racial discrimination against doctors from ethnic minorities", *British Medical Journal*, **306**, 691.

Ewles L and Simnett I (1992) *Promoting Health: A Practical Guide to Health Education*, London, Scutari Press.

Freidson E (1986) *Professional Powers: A Study of the Institutionalization of Formal Knowledge*, Chicago, University of Chicago Press.

Helman C (1986) "Feed a cold, starve a fever", in Currer C and Stacey M (eds) *Concepts of Health, Illness and Disease: A Comparative Perspective*, pp. 213–231, Leamington Spa, Berg.

Herzlich C (1973) *Health and Illness*, London, Academic Press.

d'Houtaud A and Field M (1986) "New research on the image of health", in Currer C and Stacey M (eds) *Concepts of Health, Illness and Disease: A Comparative Perspective*, pp. 235–255, Leamington Spa, Berg.

Illich I (1975) *Medical Nemesis, part 1*, London, Calder and Boyers.

Lewis G (1986) "Concepts of health and illness in a Sepik society", in Currer C and Stacey M (eds) *Concepts of Health, Illness and Disease: A Comparative Perspective*, pp. 119–135, Leamington Spa, Berg.

Lock S (1986) "Self-help groups: the fourth estate in medicine?", *British Medical Journal*, **293**, 1596–600.

Mansfield K (1977) in Stead CK (ed), *The Letters and Journals of Katherine Mansfield: A selection*, Harmondsworth, Penguin.

McKeown T (1979) *The Role of Medicine*, Basil Blackwell, Oxford. Reprinted in Black N (1984) *Health and Disease*, Milton Keynes, Open University Press.

McKeown T and Lowe CR (1974) *An Introduction to Social Medicine*, Oxford, Blackwell Scientific Publications.

National Forum for Coronary Heart Disease Prevention (1990) *CHD Prevention in Undergraduate Medical Education*, London, National Forum for Coronary Heart Disease Prevention.

Open University U205 Health and Disease Course Team (1985) Book 3: The Health of Nations, Milton Keynes, Open University Press.

Parsons T (1972) "Definitions of health and illness in the light of American values and social structure", in Jaco E and Gartley E (eds) *Patients, Physicians and Illness: A Sourcebook in Behavioural Science and Health*, pp. 97–117 London, Collier-Macmillan.

Pfeffer N (1985) "The hidden pathology of the male reproductive system", in Homans H (ed.) *The Sexual Politics of Reproduction*, Aldershot, Gower.

Rose P (ed.) (1993) *Social Trends 23 (1992)*, London, HMSO.

Seedhouse D (1986) *Health: Foundations for Achievement*, John Wiley and Sons.

Skellington R and Morris P (1992) *Race in Britain Today*, London, Sage.

Skrabanek P and McCormick J (1992) *Follies and Fallacies in Medicine*, Tarragon Press.

Stacey M (1988) *The Sociology of Health and Healing*, London, Unwin Hyman,

Townsend P, Davidson N and Whitehead M (1988) *Inequalities in Health: The Black Report and the Health Divide*, Harmondsworth, Penguin.

Williams RGA (1983) "Concepts of health: an analysis of lay logic", *Sociology*, **17**, 183–205.

Wilkinson RG (1992) "Income distribution and life expectancy", *British Medical Journal*, **304**, 165–168.

Wilson M (1975) *Health is for People*, Darton, Longman and Todd.

World Health Organisation (1946) *Constitution*, Geneva, WHO.

World Health Organisation (1984) *Health Promotion: A Discussion Document on the Concept and Principles*, Copenhagen, WHO Regional Office for Europe.

World Health Organisation (1986) "Ottawa charter for health promotion", *Journal of Health Promotion* **1**, 1–4.

2 Influences on health

Overview

The previous chapter showed there is a wide range of meanings attached to the concept of health, and different perspectives offered by the scientific medical model and social science. It emphasized the importance of social factors in the construction and meaning of health. This chapter shows how the major influences on mortality and morbidity are social and environmental factors. It summarizes recent research which suggests that there are inequalities in health status between groups of people which reflect structural inequalities in society such as social class, gender and ethnicity.

Key Points
■ Factors influencing health
■ Links between: social class and health; gender and health; and ethnicity and health
■ Effects of income, housing and employment on health
■ Explanations for health inequalities

Determinants of health

Since the decline in infectious diseases in the 19th and early 20th centuries, the major causes of sickness and death are now cardiovascular (now accounting for nearly 48% of deaths), and cancers (now accounting for 25% of deaths) (Jacobson *et al.*, 1991). Increased longevity and the current life span of women to 79 years and men to 73 years accounts for the increase in degenerative diseases in the population as a whole. However, epidemiologists who study the pattern of diseases in society have found that not all groups have the same opportunities to achieve good health and there are population patterns which make it possible to predict the likelihood that people from different groups will die prematurely.

In trying to determine what affects health, social scientists and epidemiologists will seek to compare at least two variables: firstly, a measure of health, or rather ill health, such as mortality or morbidity; and, secondly, a factor such as gender or occupation that could account for the differences in health. Of course, effects on health can be due to several variables interacting together. For example, research into coronary heart disease (CHD) has linked a large number of factors with the incidence of the disease: high levels of blood cholesterol, high blood pressure, obesity, cigarette smoking and low levels of physical activity. Other research indicates there may be links between CHD and psychosocial factors, such as stress and lack of social support, environmental factors such as hard tap water, and family history (WHO, 1982). Many studies have also tried to establish whether there is a coronary-prone personality (known as Type A) (Marmot, 1980). We also know that mortality from CHD is higher among lower social classes, among men rather than women, and among minority ethnic groups (Rose and Marmot, 1981). Figure 2.1 illustrates in a simple form how health status can be accounted for not by one variable, but by many factors which interact together. It shows that some factors have an independent effect on health or they may be mediated by other intervening variables.

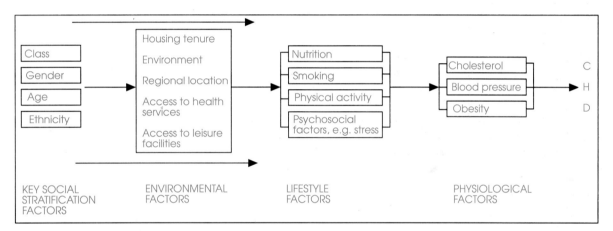

Figure 2.1 Factors influencing the development of coronary heart disease (CHD).

What is clear is that ill health does not happen by chance or through bad luck. We can group the factors which affect health into:

- Genetic factors which determine an individual's predisposition to disease
- Biological factors in which disease is caused by bacteria or viruses
- Lifestyle factors in which health behaviours such as smoking contribute to disease
- Environmental factors such as housing or pollution
- Social factors connected with the membership of particular social groups (class, gender, ethnicity, age) which may influence the other factors.

Genetic factors are largely given and what limited scope there is for intervention lies in the medical field. The previous chapter outlined McKeown's work (1979) which showed that medical interventions in the form of vaccination had remarkably little impact on mortality rates. This suggests that factors other than the purely biological determine health and well-being. Lifestyles or health behaviours are frequently offered as explanations for current health problems but, as we shall see, these are shaped and constrained by a range of social factors.

> **?** The following diagram (Figure 2.2) shows a whole range of factors or influences on smoking behaviour. You will see that some of these are social and some are environmental influences. Take another of the factors implicated in coronary heart disease such as nutrition and identify the influences on that health behaviour.

Figure 2.2 Influences on smoking behaviour.

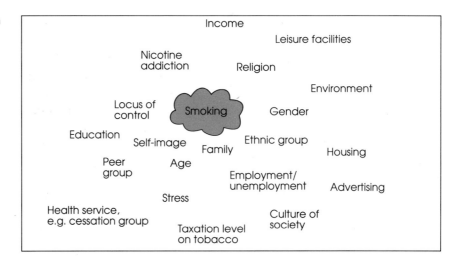

Social class and health

Most research which has sought to identify the major determinants of health and ill health has focused on the links between social class and health. In 1980 a report was published of a Department of Health and Social Security working group on inequalities in health (Townsend and Davidson, 1982). The report which is known as the Black Report after the group's chairman, Sir Douglas Black, provided a detailed study of the relationship between mortality and morbidity, and social class.

The terms social class, socio-economic status and occupation are often used interchangeably. Social class derives from the Registrar General's scale of five occupational classes ranging from professionals in class 1 to unskilled manual workers in class 5.

Because people are allocated to social classes on the basis of occupation, the classification is more suited to men of working age than the elderly or the unemployed. Married women are allocated to the social class of their husbands and therefore not properly represented either. As an indicator of social status, social class must be treated with some caution. However, class is not simply a classification of occupation but also serves as an indicator of the way of life and the living standards experienced by different groups. It correlates with other aspects of social position such as income, housing, education and working and living environments.

The main findings of the Black Report were:

- At every stage of life those in lower social classes had higher death rates than those at the top of the social scale
- Children born into the lower social classes had lower birth weights and a shorter stature
- All the major diseases affected social classes 4 and 5 more than social classes 1 and 2.

A later report commissioned by the Health Education Authority (Whitehead, 1988) confirmed many of these findings and found that the class differentials in health were becoming more marked and that other aspects of disadvantage such as unemployment and housing were also having an effect on health. More recent studies have used more complex indicators of social class and have also found marked health inequalities (Davey Smith *et al.*, 1990; Phillimore *et al.*, 1994).

Table 2.1 Social class differences in mortality rates among adults (standardized mortality ratios)* 15–64 years in England and Wales.

Social class		1959–1963		1970–1972		1979–80	1982–83†
		Men	Women	Men	Women	Men	Women
I	Professional	76	77	77	82	66	75
II	Intermediate	81	83	81	87	76	83
IIIN	Skilled non-manual	} 100	103	104	109	106	107
IIIM	Skilled manual						
IV	Semi-skilled	103	105	114	119	} 129	} 133
V	Unskilled	143	141	137	135		

* Standardized mortality ratio (SMR) is the age-adjusted death rate as a percentage of the average (100).

† Great Britain age 20–64, 20–59 for women.

Source: OPCS, *Decennial Supplements on Mortality 1971, 1978, 1986*, London HMSO.

Table 2.1 shows that mortality rates are consistently higher for social classes 4 and 5 for both men and women. Men aged 20–64 from social class 5 have more than twice the chance of dying prematurely than men in social class 1. Infant mortality is a good indicator of a country's standard of living and level of health care.

In 1984 England and Wales were ninth out of 14 European nations. Figure 2.3 shows that in 1987 a child in social class 5 was twice as likely to die before their first birthday compared to a child in social class 1 or 2. Although it is common to talk about "diseases of affluence", such as coronary heart disease and cancers, being the major killers in contemporary Britain, Figure 2.4 shows that most disease categories are more common in social classes 4 and 5. People from the lower social classes also experience more sickness and ill health. The General Household Survey each year reports that men and women from social classes 4 and 5 experience more 'limited long-standing illness' than people in social classes 1 and 2. As well as this difference in premature mortality rates between the top and bottom of the social scale, the gap in mortality rates between social class 1 and 5 has widened in the post-war period, despite a free health service and a rise in absolute and relative living standards (Wilkinson, 1986).

Although there is a clear pattern linking social class and health, there is no consensus about what it is about social class which is the most important factor. Those factors most commonly cited are income, housing or employment.

Figure 2.3 Occupational class and mortality in infants (less than 1 year) 1987 England and Wales. Source: OPCS (1987), *Mortality Statistics: Perinatal and Infant; Social and Biological Factors*, London, HMSO.

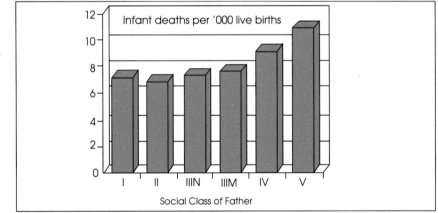

Income and health

Several reports have shown how income is a major determinant of standard of living and that variations in ill health and premature mortality reflect differences in levels of income and material deprivation (Wilkinson, 1986; British Medical Association, 1987; Townsend *et al.*, 1988). Lack of money may affect the quantity and quality of resources that can be bought. For example, low-income households tend to eat less fruit and vegetables and more refined foods higher in fat and sugar.

When money is short, food becomes a flexible item in the budget and mothers, in particular, may do without (Charles and

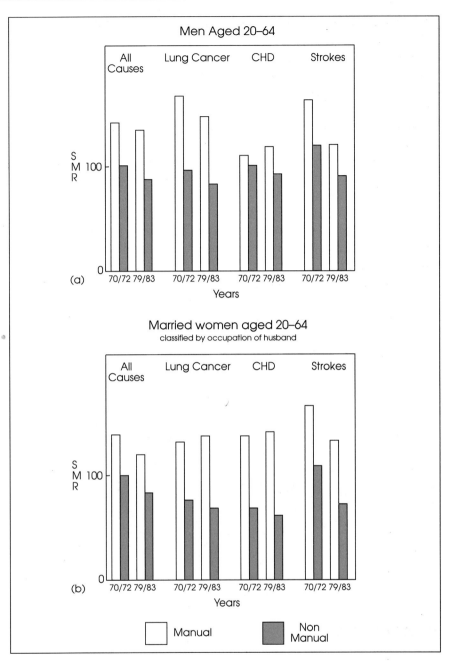

Figure 2.4
Standardized mortality ratios (SMRs) for selected causes of death in Great Britain 1970–1972 and 1979–1983 for manual and non-manual groups. (a) Men aged 20–64; (b) married women aged 20–64, classified by occupation of husbands □, manual; ■, non-manual.

Kerr, 1986; Cole-Hamilton and Lang, 1986). Income determines the type of housing in which people live. Social support and close relationships are thought to be protective of health. Social-class differences in income, and access to a car and a telephone can restrict mobility and social life. Other health effects of poverty are psychosocial and come from the stress of struggling to get by. Based on DHSS figures in 1987, 10% of the population were living on or below Income Support level and a total of 18.5 million (a third of the population) were living on the margins of poverty at 140% of that level. These are most likely to be the unemployed, pensioners, single parents, and families with three or more children.

Housing and health

Those on low incomes are more likely to be living in inadequate housing conditions, including overcrowding, damp, disrepair, and a lack of toilet, bath or cooking facilities (Whitehead, 1988). Children living in damp houses are likely to have higher rates of respiratory illness, symptoms of infection and stress (Martin *et al.*, 1987) These will be exacerbated by overcrowding. The high accident rates to children in social class 5 are associated with high density housing where there is a lack of play space and opportunities for parental supervision. Psychological and practical difficulties accompany living in high-rise flats and isolated housing estates which may adversely affect the health of women at home or older people. Another major problem is homelessness. In 1990, local authorities accepted 146,000 housing applications from homeless people. Estimates of "concealed homelessness" are put at 156,000 (Jacobson, *et al.*, 1991). The particular health problems of homelessness which include depression, high rates of infections among children and accidents, and the difficulties in gaining access to health services have been well documented (British Medical Association, 1989).

Employment and health

Particular types of employment carry high occupational health risks perhaps because of the risk of accidents, for example, in mining, exposure to hazardous substances or because of stress. Some occupations encourage lifestyles which may be damaging to health. Publicans, for example, are at high risk of developing cirrhosis.

 Consider how the following differences between manual and non-manual occupations can influence health:

■ Pay
■ Hours of work
■ Occupational pension and sickness scheme
■ Holiday entitlements
■ Accidents at work
■ Exposure to toxic substances and environmental hazards
■ Job security

(cont.)
■ Occupational mobility
■ Prestige and status
■ Autonomy.

'In the factory where I work, the women do overtime and work on Saturdays, otherwise they would not get their money, because the wage is so low and they need to make ends meet.'

'Although there was oil and grease all over the machines, washing facilities were poor. There was one toilet with cold water just in a zinc shed outside.'

'You needed a lot of concentration, because if you did not put the metal properly in the press you would break the machine. At the same time you had to go with the speed, because it was piece–work and if you didn't do it at the necessary rate you got the sack.'

Source: Mitchell, 1984.

There is also a considerable body of evidence that unemployment can damage health (Smith, 1987), although it is far from clear whether unemployment itself can lead to a deterioration in health or whether it is mediated by another variable, such as poverty, which is known to be associated with both.

? **Consider the following evidence concerning the effects of unemployment on health. What could account for this relationship?**

1. The unemployed report higher rates of mental ill health.
2. Suicide and parasuicide rates are twice as high among the unemployed as the employed.
3. The death rates among the unemployed are at least 20% higher than expected after adjustment for social class and age.
4. The unemployed have higher rates of bronchitis and ischaemic heart disease than the employed.
5. Over 60% of unemployed people smoke compared to 30% of employed people.

It seems that unemployment has a profound effect on mental health, damaging a person's self-esteem and social structure. Part of its effect on health must also arise from the material disadvantage of living on a low income.

Source: Smith, 1987.

Gender and health

Gender refers to the social categorization of people as men or women, and the social meaning and beliefs about sexual difference.

> **?** **Consider the following evidence of gender differences in health.**
>
> - Women live on average 6 years longer than men and yet women record higher levels of morbidity in both chronic and acute illness.
> - Women account for 51% of the population in the United Kingdom but account for between 60% and 65% of NHS expenditure.
> - Over 60% of general practice consultations involve women.
> - Over 60% of hospital beds are occupied by women.
> - Admissions to psychiatric hospitals have been three times higher for women than for men for most disorders.
>
> Source: Miles, 1991; Wells, 1987.

Some of the sex differences in morbidity have been attributed as an artefact of measurement of the use of health services. Women are more likely to report illness as they are less likely to be in full-time employment or because they are more inclined to take care of their health resulting in increased consultation rates. However, this does not explain the sex difference in mortality.

The natural selection or genetic explanation suggests that women are more resistant to infection and benefit from a protective effect from oestrogen accounting for their lower mortality rates. Paradoxically, female hormones and the female reproductive system are claimed to render women more liable to physical and mental ill health. Biological explanations are unable to account for the social class difference in women's health whereby women in social-class 1 and 2 experience better health than women in social classes 4 and 5.

Lifestyle explanations argue that women are socialized to be passive, dependent and sick. Women readily adopt the sick role because it fits with preconceived notions of feminine behaviour. Men, by contrast, are encouraged to be aggressive and risk-taking both at work and in their leisure time. The higher rates for accidents and alcoholism amongst men are cited as evidence for this.

Another explanation offered by feminist sociologists is that patriarchy or male power affects women's health experience. So it is argued that the medical profession is more inclined to label women as ill. Women's biological and psychological attributes are made pathological because they are seen as inferior to those of men. Women are seen as inherently sick and frail (Ehrenreich and English, 1976).

Finally, it has been argued that women's social position as both carers and workers inside, and increasingly outside, the home is a dual burden which leads to increased stress and ill health. Forty-two per cent of the employed workforce is female and yet women receive on average two-thirds of the male wage for equal work. Most women work part-time with less security and benefits than full-time workers, and working conditions at home and in the workplace are hazardous, especially for poorer women in social classes 4 and 5 (Doyal, 1987). Employment outside the home does have a protective benefit for some women but this seems to be dependent on material circumstance.

> **?**   **Many explanations have been offered to account for women's ill health. With which of the following do you most agree?**
>
> 1. Women consult their GPs more frequently than men and so will appear to have higher morbidity.
> 2. Women acknowledge their feelings of illness.
> 3. In the same situation, a man would be told to get on with things. A woman is labelled as ill.
> 4. Many women are workers inside and outside the home and have care responsibilities.
> 5. Much of women's ill health is due to depression from their social isolation at home.
> 6. Much of women's ill health relates to their reproductive organs.
> 7. The patriarchal control of medicine has deprived women of control over natural processes such as childbearing and child rearing, producing more problems.
> 8. Women have less access to material resources than men.

Health of ethnic minorities

Race is another way in which social and health inequalities are structured. This should be understood as a political and not a biological category. We therefore use the term "ethnic minority" to identify those who share a cultural heritage and who also share an experience of discrimination.

There are overall higher mortality and morbidity rates among ethnic minority groups. Findings from the Immigrant Mortality Study (Marmot *et al.*, 1984) found higher than average rates for tuberculosis and accidents, but lower than average rates for bronchitis and cancer in these groups. There was strikingly high mortality from hypertension and strokes among those from the Caribbean and African Commonwealth. Mortality statistics show disturbingly high infant mortality rates for babies born to mothers from other countries, especially Pakistan.

Professional and public attention has tended to focus not on this association between ethnicity and ill health, but on the tiny minority of ill health which can be attributed to diseases specific to certain ethnic minority groups such as sickle cell anaemia, thalassaemia and Tay–Sachs disease.

There is still very little information on the health of ethnic minorities. Until 1991 ethnic origin was not recorded in census information or official statistics. The country of birth recorded on birth and death certificates has therefore formed the basis for the association between health and ethnic origin. This clearly does not account for British-born ethnic minorities. It is important then not to put all members of ethnic minorities into one disadvantaged category. More data would enable us to find out how many people from ethnic minority groups are disadvantaged, and how. It would also then be possible to determine whether poor health is associated with the low income, poor working conditions or unemployment, and poor housing shared by those in lower social classes, or whether there is, in addition, ill health resulting from institutionalized discrimination in health care and other services (McNaught, 1987).

> **?**
>
> **Consider the following possible explanations for the high rates of hypertension in older generation black and minority ethnic communities. Which do you consider to be the most likely explanation(s)?**
>
> - Greater consumption of saturated fats in the United Kingdom.
> - High cost of imported African, Caribbean and Asian foods.
> - Stress associated with chronic situations, such as poverty and racism.
> - Lack of exercise which is not incorporated into daily life as it is in Africa and the Caribbean.
> - Retention of excess salt because of a different climate and lifestyle.

Place of residence

The Health Divide (Whitehead, 1988) shows how mortality rates increase steadily moving from the South-east to the North-west and that a North–South divide is present for most diseases, although there are significant variations *within* regions. The greatest health disparities are in regions with the poorest mortality rates – the North, Wales, Scotland and the North-west (Townsend, 1988). One obvious explanation for the geographic differences in death rates might be differences in social class distribution, those areas with high mortality rates being those areas with a greater proportion of people in social classes 4 and 5. Yet the regional mortality differences remain even after adjustment for social class and people in each social class do better in the healthier regions. Although a North–South divide does exist, it is not clear cut. The healthiest areas of the North compare favourably with those in the South.

Explaining health inequalities

We have seen that there are inequalities in health relating to social class, geographic location, gender and ethnic origin.

What explanation would you offer for the inequalities in health between social classes?

You may believe that people in the lower social classes choose more unhealthy ways of living, or you may believe that people in social classes 4 and 5 have low incomes which prevent them adopting a healthy lifestyle and cause them to live in unhealthy conditions. There is a continuing debate over this question and no simple answer. Explanations have tended to be of four broad types: artefact, social selection, cultural/behavioural and materialist/structural.

Health inequalities as an artefact

The artefact explanation argues that the widening gap in mortality figures between the social classes is not real, but an effect of the way in which class and health are measured. Because there have been changes in the classification of occupations and in the structure of social classes, it makes it impossible to make comparisons over time. For example, the assignment of occupations to social classes has changed over several decades as has the relative size of the classes. There is now a much smaller proportion of the population in class 5 and comparisons between class 1 and class 5 over 30–50 years are not comparing similar-sized segments of the population. There may have been changes in the relative status of the classes also. The smaller class 1 before 1945 may be very different from the expanded class 1 in the 1980s when the Black Report was published. It is also argued that the mortality rates of class 5 are skewed because, as social mobility continues, this class contains a greater proportion of older people at risk from dying.

Establishing a relationship between social class and health, particularly over time, is difficult. However, a considerable amount of research supports the view that the relationship is a real phenomenon and not merely an artefact of the data. When other indicators of disadvantage are used such as housing, access to a car, education, household possessions and income, they all show a similar pattern of health inequalities between the top and bottom of the social scale (Goldblatt, 1990).

Health inequalities as a selection process

Social selection theory argues that the relationship between class and health is a causal one, but that it is health which determines people's class and not vice versa. The healthy experience upward social mobility and mortality rates are kept low in the upper classes. People with higher levels of illness drift down the social scale and thus inflate the rates of death and disability among social classes 4 and 5. There is some evidence that health can affect social status. A study of women in Aberdeen found that those who were taller tended to marry into a higher social class. As height may be taken as an indicator of health, this evidence suggests some sort of health selection taking place at marriage (Illsley, 1986). Chronic illness can also account for downward social mobility. Manual workers with failing health are often moved into other jobs because of sickness and are more likely to have difficulty finding new work.

The argument suggests that health is a static property rather than a shifting state of being which is influenced by social and economic circumstance. Thus some people, because of their genetic health potential, are able to overcome disadvantage and 'climb out of poverty'. Whilst this may be true for some people, the extent of social mobility is not sufficient to account for the overall scale of social-class differences in health (Wilkinson, 1986).

Health inequalities as a result of lifestyles

This argument suggests that the social distribution of ill health is linked with differences in risk behaviours. These behaviours – smoking, high alcohol consumption, lack of exercise, high fat and sugar diets – are more common among lower social classes.

Table 2.2 shows the distribution of smoking among the social classes. It shows that while smoking has decreased in all social classes over the last two decades, there are still major differences in the proportion of smokers in classes 1 to 5. From 1972 to 1988 smoking among social classes 1 and 2 fell by 50%, while the proportion of smokers in class 5 fell by only 33%.

Table 2.2 Proportion of smokers by social class 1972 and 1988.

	1	2	3 Non-manual	3 Manual	4	5	All
Men							
1972	33	44	45	57	57	64	52
1988	16	26	25	39	40	43	33
Women							
1972	33	38	38	47	42	42	42
1988	17	26	27	35	37	39	30

Source: OPCS (1990) Monitor SS 90/2.

Wilkinson (1986) has argued that the current distribution of coronary heart disease, stroke and lung cancer and the so-called "diseases of affluence" among the lower social classes is a result of the downward social shift in the consumption of tobacco and refined foods.

Health inequalities and cultural explanations

Some writers claim that there are cultural differences between social groups in their attitudes towards health and protecting their health for the future. Thus giving up cigarettes, as a form of deferred gratification, is more likely to appeal to middle-class people whom, as we saw in Chapter 1, may have a stronger locus of control and may believe that they determine the course of their life. Working-class people who may have to struggle to get by each day do not make long-term plans and have a fatalistic view of health, believing it to be a matter of luck. Thus attitudes are passed on from generation to generation. This phenomenon is referred to as the "culture of poverty" or "cycle of deprivation". The view was summed up by Sir (now Lord) Keith Joseph, who as Minister for Health and Social Security, remarked in 1972 that inadequate people tend to be inadequate parents, and inadequate parents tend to rear inadequate children and, therefore, such people should be compulsorily sterilized.

A behavioural explanation which sees lifestyles and cultural influences determining health has considerable appeal to a Government which is concerned to reduce public expenditure. If individuals are seen as responsible for their own health, Government inactivity is legitimized. In 1986, Edwina Currie, a newly appointed health minister, caused a storm of controversy by suggesting that the high levels of premature death, permanent sickness and low birthweights in the Northern regions were due to ignorance and people failing to realize that they had some control over their lives. Views such as Currie's individualize failure by identifying problems in the home environment, and not in the social and economic conditions in which people live. Such viewpoints have been widely criticized as victim blaming, in that people are seen as being responsible for factors which disadvantage them but over which they have no control.

Cultural explanations of behaviour may be seen as an extension of individual victim blaming to cultural victim blaming – attitudes and behaviour which is different and may be perfectly rational is seen as in some way socially deficient. The working class are viewed as ignorant, feckless or too apathetic to do anything about changing their lives.

 "The problem of infant mortality is not one of sanitation alone, or housing or, indeed, of poverty as such, but is mainly a question of motherhood . . . death in infancy is probably more due to such ignorance and negligence than any other cause" (George Newman, Chief Medical Officer, 1906).

Hilary Graham (1992) has shown how the decision to smoke by many working-class women is a coping strategy to deal with the stress associated with poverty and isolation. The decision to smoke *is* a choice but it is not taken through recklessness or ignorance, but rather a choice between "health evils" – stress versus smoking.

Do you agree with those people who say that people who die from lung cancer caused by smoking have only themselves to blame?
Now consider these extracts from interviews with lone parents who have made a positive choice to smoke because it allows them to cope with parenting in adverse circumstances.

"Sometimes I put him outside the door and put the radio on at full blast, then I've sat down and had a cigarette, calmed down and fetched him in again."
"If I was economizing I'd cut down on cigarettes but I wouldn't give them up. I'd stop eating. That sounds terrible doesn't it? Food just isn't that important to me, but having a cigarette is the one thing I do for myself".'
Source: Graham 1992.

Health inequalities as a result of material disadvantage

This explanation argues that the distribution of health and ill health in the population reflects a profoundly unequal distribution of resources in society. Thus those who experience ill health are those who are lower in the social hierarchy, who are least educated, who have least money and have fewest resources. Low income may be the result of unemployment or ill-paid hazardous occupations; it can lead to poor housing in polluted and unsafe environments with few opportunities to build social support networks; and in turn such conditions lead to poor health. Lack of money can make it difficult for households to implement what they may know to be healthy choices. Blaxter (1990), analysing data from the largest health and lifestyle survey completed in the UK, found that the health of low-income groups improves substantially as income increases.

It is this explanation which the *Black Report* and *The Health Divide* adopted. The *Black Report* made 37 recommendations which comprised a comprehensive anti-poverty strategy which would reduce the health disadvantage of the working classes through improved welfare benefits, housing programmes, better working conditions and income redistribution through taxation.

Marxist sociologists have suggested that the patterns of health in society reflect the way in which society itself is structured. Thus the economic inequalities of a capitalist economic system are implicated directly or indirectly as a cause of illness. Doyal and Pennell (1979) suggest that the capitalist mode of production damages health in the following ways.

(cont.)

1. Occupational health hazards such as pollution, noise, dangerous machinery and unsafe working practices.
2. The effects on mental health from alienating work.
3. The destruction of social relationships based on community through the need for a mobile labour force.
4. The periods of boom and slump associated with capitalism cause periodic unemployment with its attendant threats to mental health.
5. The promotion of products such as tobacco, alcohol, processed foods and powdered baby milk. These commodities pose a health risk because they are highly processed, the result of modern methods of production. Their consumption is promoted through mass advertising not because they are useful but because they have higher profit margins.

Access to health services

The inequalities in health that we have considered in this chapter are all the more remarkable because the National Health Service has been in existence for more than 40 years. Its intention to provide a universal service freely available to all might have been expected to reduce inequalities in health status. Yet in the early 1970s a GP writing in *The Lancet* put forward a radical view that good health care tends to vary inversely with the need of the population (Tudor Hart, 1971).

 "In areas with most sickness and death, GPs have more work, larger lists, less hospital support and inherit more clinically ineffective traditions of consultation than in the healthiest areas; and the hospital doctors shoulder heavier caseloads with less staff and equipment, more obsolete buildings and suffer recurrent crises in the availability of beds and replacement of staff. These trends can be summed up as the Inverse Care Law: that the availability of good medical care tends to vary inversely with the needs of the population served."

 Consider the following evidence cited by Whitehead (1988) of differences in health care.

The World Health Organisation (1985) declared that, in health care, social justice should lead to "equal access to available care, equal treatment for equal cases and equal quality of care". Yet several studies have found that opportunities to obtain quality in health care are not equal. Working-class areas have more single-handed practices and GPs in these areas tend to be older (compulsory retirement at 70 was recommended in the White Paper "Promoting Better Health"). The quality of care is also different. Middle-class patients tend to have longer consultations, more opportunity to discuss their problems, and are better known by their GPs (Cartwright and O'Brien, 1976). In addition there is a clear class gradient in attendance at antenatal clinic, child health clinics, cervical screening and dental health services.

What reasons can you offer for the low take up of preventive services by working class people?

Some of the reasons may relate to ease of access. Working-class and older people who do not have cars may find public transport difficult, especially those with young children. Clinics may lack play space. For hourly paid workers, attendance at primary health care clinics may mean loss of earnings. The use of appointment systems by clinics and GP surgeries causes difficulties for households without a telephone. There is also evidence that health care workers respond differently to different social groups. Thus working-class people may have low expectations of primary health care. Or is the most likely explanation to do with cultural attitudes? As discussed earlier in this chapter, some writers suggest that working-class people do not value their health and have a fatalistic attitude towards prevention.

There is evidence of variation in the quality and quantity of care available to people in different social groups, between regions and between different ethnic groups. However, since medical care has had little impact on the overall death rate from heart disease or cancers, and probably only about 5% deaths are preventable through medical treatment, it must be concluded that differences in health status are not wholly attributable to variations in the amount and type of care received.

Conclusion

Health promotion is not a purely technical activity. As we have seen, even identifying the causes of ill health will lead to political judgements being made.

Consider the following points of view about the causes of health and illness. Which comes closest to your own?

■ Ill health is the result of people's unhealthy lifestyles. No one makes people live this way and so it is up to individuals to take responsibility for their own health. The role of the health promoter is to provide information to encourage people to be concerned about their health and make healthier decisions.
■ Ill health is the result of the social and economic conditions in which people live. It is not a person's fault if they become ill. People may have unhealthy lifestyles but this is because it is difficult to make healthy choices on a low income. The role of the health promoter is to try to empower people to take charge of their lives by raising awareness of the factors that influence their health. Health promoters need to draw the attention of policy makers to the influence of social and economic conditions on their clients' health.

In any area of work or discipline, there will always be debate about what constitutes good practice. It is important to clarify your thinking and where you stand because it will affect your views on the purpose of health promotion and what would be appropriate health promotion activities. It is also important that you share these thoughts with colleagues and clients to reach a common understanding of the ideals upon which health promotion activities are based.

In practice, behavioural and structural explanations are often aligned to the right or left of the political spectrum, and have become linked with very different policies and approaches to health promotion. The behavioural approach which focuses on individual lifestyles has informed much of health education because it suggests that information, advice or mass media messages can change behaviours such as smoking or sexual activity. A structural approach which sees health as determined by social and economic conditions, and reflecting the unequal distribution of power and resources in society, requires the health promoter to become involved in political activity.

Many health promoters may find it difficult to acknowledge economic and social determinants of health in their practice. The Health of the Nation strategy (Department of Health, 1992) stops short of identifying these fundamental causes of ill health, with poverty failing to be mentioned once. Health promoters may also feel powerless to effect change on such a fundamental level. Yet it is possible to identify small changes in practice which give more regard to social conditions. For example, the Health Visitors Association annual conference in 1992 identified a key role in:

  Identifying clients' own considered needs
  Speaking out on behalf of individuals, families and communities suffering poverty and deprivation
  Arguing for more resources
  Identifying poverty as a factor in caseload profiles
  Providing a health and social commentary for managers and policy makers (Blackburn, 1992).

Questions for further discussion

  Is it fair or effective to encourage individuals to change their health behaviour?
  Good health depends on adequate income. Do you agree?
  What long-term social policy initiatives would most bring about an improvement in the health of your clients?
  What are the implications for professional practice of the links between health and wealth?

Summary

This chapter has reviewed the evidence concerning health differences in the population and the physical, social and environmental variables that are implicated in ill health: poverty, unemployment, inadequate housing, stressful and dangerous working conditions, lack of social support, air and water pollution. It goes on to consider the ways in which risk factors associated with personal behaviour – smoking, nutrition, exercise – are influenced by the social environment.

Several explanations for inequalities in health have been discussed. None offers a complete explanation, but the chapter concludes that there is sufficient evidence to point to social and economic factors determining health. It argues that disadvantage can give rise to or exacerbate health-damaging behaviours such as smoking or poor nutrition, and so health behaviours should not be separated from their social context.

Further reading

Association of Community Health Councils (1990) *Health and Wealth: A Review of Health Inequalities in the UK*, London, Association of Community Health Councils.

A useful, concise summary of the arguments relating to health inequalities summarizing evidence on social class; income; diet and health and housing and health.

Townsend P, Davidson N and Whitehead M (1992) *Inequalities in Health*, 2nd edn, London, Penguin.

The Black Report and The Health Divide published in one volume. The most significant reports on health status and still essential reading.

Jacobson B, Smith A and Whitehead M (1991) *The Nation's Health: A Strategy for the 1990s*, 2nd edn, London, King's Fund.

An accessible and readable assessment of trends in health status and public health policy over the last decade. A detailed analysis is offered of income, employment, housing and nutrition as well as aspects of lifestyle such as tobacco, alcohol consumption and exercise.

References

Blackburn C (1992) *Improving Health and Welfare Work with Families in Poverty: A Handbook*, Milton Keynes, Open University Press.

Blaxter M (1990) *Health and Lifestyles*, London, Routledge.

British Medical Association (1987) *Deprivation and Health*, London, BMA Board of Science and Education.

British Medical Association (1989) *Homeless Families and their Health*, London, HVA and General Medical Services Committee.

Cartwright A and O'Brien M (1976) "Social class variations in health care", in Stacey M (1976) (ed.) *The Sociology of the NHS*, Sociological Review Monograph 22, University of Keele.

Charles N and Kerr M (1986) "Issues of responsibility and control in the feeding of families", in Rodmell S and Watt A (eds) *The Politics of Health Education*, London, Routledge and Kegan Paul.

Cole-Hamilton I and Lang T (1986) *Tightening Belts: A Report on the Impact of Poverty on Food*, London, London Food Commission

Davey Smith G, Bartley M and Blane D (1990) "The Black Report on socio-economic inequalities in health ten years on", *British Medical Journal*, **301**, 373–375

Department of Health (1992) *The Health of the Nation*, London, HMSO.

Doyal L (1987) Unhealthy Lives: *Being a Woman in London*, Womens Study Unit, Polytechnic of North London.

Doyal L and Pennell I (1979) *The Political Economy of Health*, London, Pluto,

Ehrenreich B and English D (1976) *Complaints and Disorders: The Sexual Politics of Sickness*, London, Writers and Readers Publishing Cooperative.

Goldblatt P (1990) *Longitudinal Study: Mortality and Social Organisation 1971-81 England and Wales*, OPCS Series LS No 8. London, HMSO.

Graham H (1992) *Smoking Among Working Class Mothers with Children*, Department Applied Social Studies, University of Warwick.

Illsley R (1986) "Occupational class, selection, and the production of inequalities", *Quarterly Journal of Social Affairs*, **2** (2), 151–165.

Jacobson B, Smith A and Whitehead M (1991) *The Nation's Health*, London, King's Fund.

Marmot MG (1980) "Type A personality and ischemic heart disease", *Psychological Medicine*, **10**, 603–606

Marmot MG, Adelstein AM and Bulusu L (1984) Immigrant

Mortality in England and Wales 1970–1978, OPCS Studies on Medical and Population Subjects No 47, London, HMSO.

Martin CJ, Platt SD and Hunt SM (1987) "Housing and ill health", *British Medical Journal*, **294**, 1125–1127.

McKeown T (1979) *The Role of Medicine: Dream Mirage or Nemesis*, Oxford, Blackwell.

McNaught A (1987) *Health Action and Ethnic Minorities*, London, Bedford Square Press.

Miles A (1991) *Women, Health and Medicine*, Milton Keynes, Open University.

Mitchell J (1984) *What is to be Done about Illness and Health?*, London, Penguin.

OPCS (1990) Cigarette smoking 1972–1988. OPCS Monitor SS 90/2.

Phillimore P, Beattie A and Townsend P (1994) "Widening inequality of health in northern England", *British Medical Journal*, **308**, 1125–1128.

Rose G and Marmot MG (1981) "Social class and coronary heart disease", *British Heart Journal*, **45**, 13–19.

Smith R (1987) *Unemployment and Health*, Oxford, Oxford University Press.

Townsend P and Davidson N (1982) *Inequalities in Health: the Black Report*, London, Penguin.

Townsend P, Phillimore P and Beattie A (1988) *Health and Deprivation: Inequalities and the North*, London, Routledge.

Tudor Hart J (1971) "The inverse care law", *Lancet*, **i**, 405.

Wells N (1987) *Womens Health Today*, London, Office of Health Economics.

Whitehead M (1988) *The Health Divide*, London, Health Education Council.

Wilkinson RG (ed.) (1986) *Class and Health: Research and Longtitudinal Data*, London, Tavistock.

World Health Organisation (1982) *Prevention of Coronary Heart Disease, Report of a WHO Expert Committee*, Technical Report Series, Geneva, WHO.

World Health Organisation (1985) *Social Justice and Equity in Health, Report from the Programme on Social Equity and Health*, Leeds, WHO.

3 Measuring health

Overview

We have seen in Chapter 1 how people define health in different ways and in Chapter 2 how there are different determinants of health. This would suggest that measuring health is not a simple task. This appears to be borne out by the existence of a number of ways of measuring health and a lack of clear agreement about which are the best ways to measure health. This chapter looks first at why we might want to measure health. It goes on to investigate the different means of measuring health currently in use and unpacks some of the assumptions underlying their use. Finally, the uses of the different kinds of measures are explored. The practical uses of measuring health are discussed further in Chapters 11 and 12 on needs assessment and programme planning, and in Chapter 13 on evaluation.

Key points
- Mortality rates
  - Standardized mortality rate
  - Infant mortality rate
  - Perinatal and neonatal mortality rate
- Morbidity rates
- Hospital activity analysis
- Health status measures
- Functional ability and disability
- Health behaviour indicators
- Environmental indicators
- Nottingham health profile
- Jarman index
- Quality of life
- QALYs
- Health targets

Why measure health?

Finding a means to measure health is an important practical task for health promoters. There are several reasons why this is so.

1. To assist planning. Health promoters need information to assist the planning and evaluation of health promotion programmes. It is important to establish baseline data in order to plan priorities and to have a standard against which health promotion interventions can be evaluated.
2. To justify resources. Health promotion is often in competition with other activities for scarce resources. To make a claim for resources and to prove that their activities are effective, health promoters need information on the health status of populations.
3. To assist the development of the profession. Measurements of health gain are important to the professional development of health promoters. Unless there is a means of measuring the effect of our actions, health promotion work will remain invisible, underfunded and low priority. By demonstrating the efficacy of health promotion interventions, it is possible to argue for resources, credibility and funding.

Depending on the purpose, different measures of health may be used or developed.

The means of measuring health depend primarily on the view of health which is held. If someone believes health is basically about physical functioning, then measures of physical fitness will be an adequate measure of health. If health is defined as having no disease, then measures of the extent of disease may be used (in reverse) as measures of health. However, if health is defined as including social and mental aspects and as meaning something other than being not ill, specific measurements of health will need to be developed.

Noack (1991) proposes a framework for conceptualizing and measuring health which includes both the time dimension (past, present and future) and the health level (individual and population) (Table 3.1). This framework yields six cells: health history, health balance and health potential, for the individual and the population.

Table 3.1 A conceptual framework for measuring health (from Noack, 1991).

Time	Concept	Level	
		Individual	Population
Past	Health history	Health balance in personal life Positive health career (growing health balance) Negative health career (declining health balance)	Stable and high level of well-being over time Increasing level of well-being over time Decreasing level of well-being over time
Present	Health balance	General well-being and functioning Social functioning and social support Psychological well-being and functioning Physical well-being and functioning	High prevalence of general well-being Social integration and mutual support High prevalence of psychological well-being High prevalence of physical well-being
Future	Health potential	Overall personal health resources Strong supportive social relations Strong, positive self-concept Life and coping skills Level of somatic risk factors Level of physical fitness	Equity of access to general health resources Life expectancy free of suffering and disability Survival and quality of life of chronically ill people Frequency of self-help activities Overall level of positive lifestyle

Note The entries are only examples that are neither representative nor exhaustive.

It is argued that this framework clarifies the kind of health measures most appropriate for specific purposes. It also emphasizes that health is a dynamic phenomenon and that any measure is a snapshot in time.

We shall look next at the different ways of measuring health, starting with the measurement of health as a negative variable and moving on to consider the measurement of health as a positive variable. Measuring health as a negative variable means measuring the opposite to health (e.g. disease or death) and using these results to infer the degree of health. Health is therefore being defined as a negative (health is not being ill or dead), not as a positive (health in its own right).

Measuring health as a negative variable (e.g. health is not being diseased or ill)

The most common means of measuring health as a negative variable are mortality and morbidity statistics. The Government and health authorities already collect a wealth of information concerning disease, illness and death rates. The Office of Population Censuses and Surveys (OPCS) is responsible for collecting a range of data. For example, the ten yearly census data covering the whole of the population provides standard demographic data such as population estimates broken down into age bands. The OPCS Monitors provide data relating to deaths broken down by cause of death and region. Statistics on the abortion rate are collected and published. Deaths around childbirth are monitored in detail, and perinatal and infant mortality rates are published. The OPCS also produces birth statistics.

There are several sources of data concerning illness rates, including the General Household Survey, the Royal College of General Practitioners and health authorities. More details on these sources of data and their shortcomings are given in the section on morbidity statistics below.

Data on deaths and illnesses are often used as surrogate measures of health. There are obviously shortcomings to this approach. Measuring conditions which limit health, such as illness, is not the same as measuring health itself. Measuring mortality rates does not provide any information about the quality of health experienced by people when they were alive.

These statistics can also be used in international comparisons because most countries hold some form of database on deaths and disease rates. Although these statistics are often presented as if they were objective facts, it is important to remember that statistics are devised by people in a social context, subject to assumptions, bias and error. At every stage of the data-collecting process, decisions are taken which help shape the ultimate form of information presented.

> **?** It is often suggested that suicide is under-reported as a cause of death. Can you think of any reasons why this might be the case?
>
> Suicide and mental illness tend to be stigmatized, that is, they have negative meanings which become attached to the person affected, their relatives and friends. Suicide may be contrary to cultural or religious beliefs, and a diagnosis of suicide as cause of death may also have repercussions in terms of insurance. For all these reasons, suicide is likely to be under-reported.

Information is generated in a social context which may also encourage and reinforce social stereotypes. For example, a common measurement used to assess the success of medical intervention is return to paid employment. This ignores the fact that opportunities for paid employment are affected by many factors other than health, such as the unemployment rate, age, gender, class and race. In particular, use of this measure ignores the fact that for many women domestic work and not paid employment is the relevant factor. Official statistics are often presented in ways which reproduce sexist assumptions about the nature of men and women (Oakley and Oakley, 1981; Roberts, 1990).

> **?** Lung cancer is a disease category listed in the International Disease Classification System (IDCS). This means lung cancer is acceptable as a cause of ill health or death. Tobacco use is not listed in the IDCS.
>
> ■ What impact do you think this has on our perception of risk factors and causes of disease, and on suitable strategies for prevention and treatment?
> ■ Is it likely to foster understanding of social, environmental or biological causes of disease?

Mortality statistics

There are several different ways of expressing death rates. The crude death rate is the number of deaths per 1000 people per year. However, this figure is obviously affected by the age structure of the population which may vary over time and region. An area with a high proportion of elderly, such as a south coast retirement town, would have consistently higher death rates than a more deprived area with a higher percentage of premature deaths, such as an inner city area. The Standardized Mortality Ratio (SMR) measures the death rate taking into account differences in age structure. The death rate of a selected population at a given time is taken as the baseline and death rates for specific age bands are calculated. The

Registrar General of England and Wales uses the mortality rate for 1950–1952 as this baseline standard in many of its publications. *The Health of the Nation* (Department of Health, 1992) document adopts 1990 as the baseline year for its health targets. The SMR for any subsequent year is then the number of deaths actually occurring as a percentage of the deaths which would have been expected to occur if the population's age-specific mortality experience had remained at its baseline level. The SMR is therefore an attempt to measure the underlying trend of death rates. The SMR is useful because it can be used for comparisons, and to judge trends.

The infant mortality rate (IMR) is another commonly used statistic. The IMR is the number of deaths in the first year of life per 1000 live births. The IMR is strongly associated with adult mortality rates, and is sensitive to changes in preventive medicine and improved health service delivery. The IMR is therefore capable of being used as an indicator of the general health of the population, particularly when comparisons between countries are being drawn. The perinatal mortality rate (PMR) is the number of stillbirths and deaths in the first 7 days after birth per 1000 births. The neonatal death rate is the number of deaths occurring in the first 28 days after birth per 1000 live births. Both the SMR and the IMR are readily available statistics, and therefore easy to use as surrogate measures of health. Table 3.2 compares the PMR and IMR for different countries in Europe.

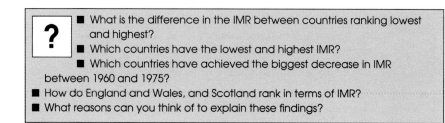

- What is the difference in the IMR between countries ranking lowest and highest?
- Which countries have the lowest and highest IMR?
- Which countries have achieved the biggest decrease in IMR between 1960 and 1975?
- How do England and Wales, and Scotland rank in terms of IMR?
- What reasons can you think of to explain these findings?

Death rates are also available broken down by gender, social class and cause. In Britain, it is well established that death rates are related to social class and gender (Townsend Davidson and Whitehead, 1988). People in the lower social classes have higher than average death rates at all ages and for virtually all causes. Women on average live longer than men, so their premature death rate is lower than that of men. This is discussed in greater detail in Chapter 2.

Reductions in mortality for selected causes among targeted groups in the population constitute the majority of the Government's "Health of the Nation" targets (Table 3.3).

Table 3.2 Perinatal and infant mortality in Europe (from Townsend et al., 1988).

	Perinatal mortality per 1000 live births				Infant mortality per 1000 live births			
	1960	1975	% decrease 1960–1975	Annual % decrease 1971–1975	1960	1975	% decrease 1960–1975	Annual % decrease 1972–1975
England and Wales	33.5	17.9*	46.5‡	4.1	21.8	14.2*	34.3‡	4.5
Scotland	38.1	18.5*	51.3‡	5.1	26.4	14.8*	44.0‡	5.4
Sweden	26.2	11.1	57.7	7.3	16.6	8.3	50.0	7.7
Norway	24.0	14.2	40.8	5.1	18.9	11.1	41.3	2.0
Denmark	26.5	12.7*	52.1‡	5.5	21.5	10.3*	52.0‡	3.9
Finland	25.3	13.9†	45.0§	5.9	21.0	11.0†	47.6§	1.4
Netherlands	25.6	14.0	45.3	4.3	16.5	10.6	35.7	3.1
France	31.8	19.5†	38.7§	4.8	27.4	11.1	59.8	10.2
West Germany	36.3	19.4	46.5	4.8	33.8	19.7	41.6	4.5
(East Germany)	—	(17.6)	—	—	—	(15.9)	—	(3.4)
USA	29.4	20.7	29.2	—	26.0	16.1	38.1	4.3

* 1976. † 1974. ‡ 1960–1976. § 1960–1974.
Sources: 1960–1972 data: Health Care – the Growing Dilemma; 1975 data: WHO and World Health Statistics, 1978, Vol.1; 1975, France: Eurohealth Handbook, 1978.

Table 3.3 Health of the Nation main targets

Coronary heart disease and stroke*

■ To reduce death rates for both CHD and stroke in people under 65 by at least 40% by the year 2000 (*Baseline 1990*)

■ To reduce the death rate for CHD in people aged 65–74 by at least 30% by the year 2000 (*Baseline 1990*)

■ To reduce the death rate for stroke in people aged 65–74 by at least 40% by the year 2000 (*Baseline 1990*)

Cancers*

■ To reduce the death rate for breast cancer in the population invited for screening by at least 25% by the year 2000 (*Baseline 1990*)

■ To reduce the incidence of invasive cervical cancer by at least 20% by the year 2000 (*Baseline 1986*)

■ To reduce the death rate for lung cancer under the age of 75 by at least 30% in men and by at least 15% in women by 2010 (*Baseline 1990*)

■ To halt the year-on-year increase in the incidence of skin cancer by 2005

Mental illness*

■ To improve significantly the health and social functioning of mentally ill people

■ To reduce the overall suicide rate by at least 15% by the year 2000 (*Baseline 1990*)

■ To reduce the suicide rate of severely mentally ill people by at least 33% by the year 2000 (*Baseline 1990*)

HIV/AIDS and sexual health

■ To reduce the incidence of gonorrhoea by at least 20% by 1995 (*Baseline 1990*), as an indicator of HIV/AIDS trends

■ To reduce by at least 50% the rate of conceptions amongst the under 16s by the year 2000 (*Baseline 1989*)

Accidents*

■ To reduce the death rate for accidents among children under 15 by at least 33% by 2005 (*Baseline 1990*)

■ To reduce the death rate for accidents among young people aged 15–24 by at least 25% by 2005 (*Baseline 1990*)

■ To reduce the death rate for accidents among people aged 65 and over by at least 33% by 2005 (*Baseline 1990*)

* The 1990 baseline for all mortality targets represents an average of the three years centred around 1990.

Why do you think sexual health is alone in not having a target which aims to reduce mortality rates?

Possible reasons include: low numbers of deaths, long time lag between preventive action and outcome of reduced mortality, and concern with morbidity rather than mortality.

■ Are any of these factors relevant?
■ Are there any other relevant factors?

Morbidity statistics

Statistics measuring illness and disease are more difficult to obtain. This is due in part to the difficulty in establishing a hard and fast line between health and disease. There is no one source of data for the whole population concerning disease and illness. Instead, there are a number of different sources of relevant information.

Notifiable infectious diseases are reported to the Communicable Disease Surveillance Centre (CDSC) who publish these statistics. Statistics on the incidence of cancer are compiled by the Cancer Registry. The health services collect routine data on the use of their services and activity rate. This data can be used to express the disease experience of different populations but there are several problems with adopting this approach.

The main problem with using many of the health authority measurements is that they were developed primarily for administrative, planning or management tasks, and reflect available services and use of these services, rather than health itself. Health authority data is primarily collected as a management tool. To some extent, this determines what data is collected. However, the advantage of using this kind of data is that it is routinely collected, is consistent across regions and is easily accessed.

> **?** Hospital activity analysis (HAA) data record episodes of treatment, not patients treated.
>
> ■ What will this data tell you about the health status of the local population?
> ■ What does it not tell you?
> ■ Why do you think it is collected in this way?

The General Household Survey (GHS) is a continuous Government survey of a sample of the population. The GHS includes questions on people's experience of illness, both long-term (chronic) and within the last fortnight (acute). GHS data is difficult to use comparatively over time as the wording of the questions changes occasionally. The following are examples of questions used in the 1990 GHS (Smyth and Brown, 1992, p. 275):

■ Over the last 12 months would you say your health has on the whole been good, fairly good or not good?
■ Do you have any long-standing illness, disability or infirmity? By long-standing I mean anything that has troubled you over a period of time or that is likely to affect you over a period of time.
■ Now I'd like you to think about the 2 weeks ending yesterday. During those 2 weeks, did you have to cut down on any of the things you usually do (about the house/at work or in your free time) because of (any chronic condition cited earlier in the interview) illness or injury?

The GHS is useful in providing information on people's subjective experience of illness, because it relies on people's self-reported illness rather than use of services.

The Government collects statistics on the number of days lost at work due to sickness. Such information is sometimes used as a measurement of morbidity. However, such data are available only for people in paid employment. The large section of the population who are not in paid employment, and their experience of illness, is therefore invisible. It is known that unemployment is associated with a marked increase in morbidity and mortality (Dhooge and Dooris, 1988).

> **?**
>
> **Two areas of equal size and population structure experience very different unemployment rates. Area A has 40% unemployment whilst Area B has 10%. The sickness rate for employed people is the same.**
>
> ■ Numerically, which area will have the greatest ill health if days lost at work due to sickness is the measure used?
> ■ Will this reflect the likely extent of ill health in the two areas?
>
> Area B will have the highest sickness rate, but it is likely that the actual extent of ill health will be greater in Area A.

Various Government research studies have developed measures to assess disability and to produce estimates of the number of people with disabilities in the population. These disability indices are based on the results of questionnaires asking people what, if any, difficulty they experience in daily life. The onus is therefore placed on the individual being unable to perform certain tasks such as bathing themselves or walking unaided up flights of stairs. The reason for these difficulties could be located in housing design and might be capable of being remedied by modifying the home environment. However, by treating disability as an inherent individual attribute, the effect of the social environment in generating and maintaining disability is rendered invisible. Abberley (1992) criticizes disability indices for reinforcing the social production of disability, by treating social factors which produce disability as given and unalterable. In this way, he argues, they fail to address the real concerns of people with disabilities.

> **?**
>
> **A typical question from disability surveys is: 'Does your health problem/disability affect your work in any way at present?'**
>
> ■ How many different reasons can you think of for someone answering 'yes' to this question?
> ■ How many of these reasons refer to physical diseases?
> ■ Mental illnesses?
> ■ Social factors?

These statistical measures of mortality, illness, disease and disability are often used to talk about health. Such usage reinforces, albeit in an indirect way, the definition of health as 'not disease'. But the advantage of such statistics is that they are already collected, are relatively consistent and are readily available. Recognizing the limitations of such measures has prompted health promoters to develop new means of measuring health as an independent phenomenon distinct from illness or disease. These measures may be conveniently divided into those describing health as an objective quality which is an attribute of people or environments, and those describing health as a subjective reality which is socially produced.

Measuring health as a positive variable

Measures of health as an objective attribute

There are a number of ways of measuring health as an objective factor including:

- Health measures
- Health behaviour indicators
- Environmental indicators
- Socio-economic indicators.

Health measures

There are measures of the health status of people, including vital statistics such as height and weight, and dental health status (the decayed, missing and filled teeth, or DMF, index). Floud (1989) argues that the average height of a population may be taken as a measure of health, as it represents a proxy for nutritional status and therefore welfare. In the same way, Townsend *et al.* (1987) use the percentage of low birthweight babies as an indicator of health.

Health behaviour indicators

Increasingly common are measurements of people's behaviour which is then used as a measure of health. For example, the number of people smoking, drinking alcohol, using drugs, taking regular exercise, eating a healthy diet, practising safer sex or planned fertility, may all be used to describe different populations, and to make comparisons between them regarding relative health status. These lifestyle measures are sometimes narrowed down to more specific behaviour in relation to the health services. For example, the percentage of children immunized against childhood illnesses, or the percentage of women screened for cervical and breast cancer, may be used to describe the health status of a population.

Environmental indicators

The same method may be applied to physical and social environments. Measurements of the physical environment include air and water quality, and housing type and density. These measures are routinely collected by the environmental health departments of local authorities.

Socio-economic indicators

The social environment may also be measured in terms of its 'healthiness'. One of the measures most commonly used to assess the social environment is wealth. Table 3.4 compares health indicators and the gross national product (GNP, a measure of a country's wealth) of different countries.

Table 3.4 Health indicators and GNP per capita for selected countries, 1980 (from Open University, 1985).

	GNP per capita, 1980 (US dollars)	Expectation of life at birth (years)	Infant mortality rate (aged 0–1)	Child death rate (aged 1–4)
Bangladesh	130	46	136	20
Sri Lanka	270	66	44	3
Sierra Leone	280	47	208	50
China	290	64	56	5
Kenya	420	55	87	15
Cuba	N/A	73	21	1
Brazil	2 050	63	77	7
South Africa	2 300	61	96	18
Portugal	2 370	71	35	2
Poland	3 900	72	21	1
USSR	4 550	71	27	1
UK	7 920	73	12	1
Saudi Arabia	11 260	54	114	18
USA	11 360	74	13	1
Sweden	13 520	75	7	0

Data from World Bank (1982, Tables 1 and 21).

> **?**
>
> **In general, the wealthier countries are those with the best health indicators. However, there are exceptions to this general trend.**
>
> ■ Can you identify these exceptions?
> ■ What might account for countries with low GNP but good health indicators?
> ■ What might account for countries with high GNP but poor health indicators?

The evidence suggests that countries with a more equitable distribution of wealth enjoy better health and that countries with very unequal distribution of wealth suffer poorer health (Open University, 1985; Wilkinson, 1992).

Objective measurements of people's health status, health-related behaviour and the environment may be combined to provide an overall picture of health. The health of different populations, from neighbourhoods to nations, may be assessed and compared using this method. Targets for improvements in health may also be set using these measurements. This is the approach adopted internationally by the WHO and nationally by the Government.

The WHO European Region's 'Health for All 2000 Targets' (WHO, 1985) and the British Government's White Paper *The Health of the Nation* (Department of Health, 1992) both list a series of targets by which improvements in health over a specific period of time may be measured. The targets include reductions in people's experience of ill health and premature mortality (e.g. reductions in accident rates and percentage of people dying prematurely from coronary heart disease), and improvements in people's health related behaviour (e.g. reduction in smoking levels, increase in percentage undertaking regular exercise).

Improvements in the social and physical environment, such as an increase in the number of smoke-free places, an increase in the number, accessibility and safety of play areas and sports centres, or improvements in housing amenities and density, may also be added in to the equation (Catford, 1983; WHO, 1985). People's health-related beliefs and attitudes, and the extent to which they conform to professional beliefs, have also been considered to be a measure of health (Catford, 1983). For example, the percentage of the population seeking to make recommended lifestyle changes, or having an understanding of basic health issues, has been suggested as a positive health measure. Combining a number of discrete elements to measure health is attractive because it gives a more rounded picture of health, and provides a clear basis and direction for health promoters.

Researchers working in Britain have developed measures of health which aggregate socio-environmental data. The Jarman index is a formula which is said to express the health needs of communities served by health authorities. The impetus for the development of these indicators was administrative; to attempt to find a fairer means of remuneration for general practitioners (GPs) serving deprived communities. The Jarman index (Jarman, 1983) combines OPCS census data with factors identified by GPs as increasing workload and pressure of work. Some factors, such as the percentage of people over 65 years in the population, were excluded because this is already included in determining levels of remuneration for GPs.

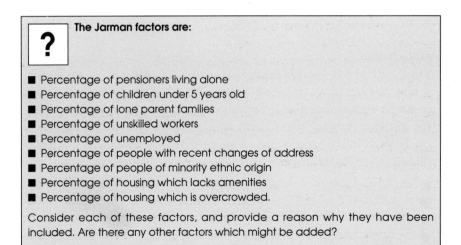

? The Jarman factors are:

- Percentage of pensioners living alone
- Percentage of children under 5 years old
- Percentage of lone parent families
- Percentage of unskilled workers
- Percentage of unemployed
- Percentage of people with recent changes of address
- Percentage of people of minority ethnic origin
- Percentage of housing which lacks amenities
- Percentage of housing which is overcrowded.

Consider each of these factors, and provide a reason why they have been included. Are there any other factors which might be added?

Measures of health as subjective reality

The previous section has outlined means of measuring health as if it were an objective property of beings, societies, or environments, capable of scientific scrutiny. However, it is apparent that health is not such a simple or uncontested attribute. Chapter 1 highlighted the importance of subjective interpretations of health and the multiple meanings health may have in different contexts. This has led some researchers to attempt to devise measurements of health which rely on subjective reporting of health. Measurements of subjective health may be broadly divided into five different types (Bowling, 1992):

- Measures of functional ability
- Broader measures of health status
- Measures of psychological well-being
- Measures of social networks and social support
- Measures of quality of life.

? **Match the following measures to the five types of health measurement given above.**

- Percentage of the population who feel they have a confidante with whom they can share things
- Percentage of the population who have restricted mobility and are unable to go outdoors without assistance
- Percentage of the population classified as obese
- Percentage of the population who report feeling content with their lives
- Percentage of the population who report feeling sad or depressed most of the time these days.

Functional ability

Measures of functional ability use people's self-reports of physical activity, such as the ability to perform everyday activities (Stewart *et al.*, 1981; Hunt, 1988). People's rating of their fitness level has also been used (Chambers *et al*, 1982).

Health status

The Nottingham Health Profile (Hunt *et al.*, 1986) is an example of a broader measure of health status. This health profile arose from research examining the most important aspects of health cited by the general public. It has been used extensively, and is claimed to be both reliable and valid. The profile consists of six separate dimensions which are scored independently. These are:

- Physical mobility
- Pain
- Sleep
- Social isolation

- Emotional reactions
- Energy level.

All of these items are scored by respondents on a standard questionnaire. The profile is therefore a subjective assessment of people's health status, and one which places equal emphasis on mental and physical health. Hunt *et al.* (1986) claim the profile is more useful as a predictor of subsequent health outcomes than more objective measurements of health status. The Nottingham Health Profile is a means of rigorously assessing health and it is increasingly being used in conjunction with other socio-environmental measures to create health profiles of areas (e.g. Department of Epidemiology and Public Health Medicine, University of Bristol Medical School, 1989).

Psychological well-being

Psychological well-being scales have measured the presence or absence of symptoms such as anxiety or depression (Dupuy, 1984). More positive measures such as happiness and life satisfaction have also been used. Life satisfaction refers to the dimension of cognition (mental state) and happiness refers to affect (feeling state). Well-being refers to both dimensions of affective well-being and cognitive functioning (McDowell and Newell, 1987). Other measures include self-esteem, a sense of coherence and perceived control over one's life. Together, these attributes have been said to constitute a psychological immune system which protects against psychological morbidity (Antonovsky 1987).

Social health

Health includes the dimension of social health, which has been defined as the degree to which people function adequately as members of the community (Renne, 1974; Greenblatt, 1975). A key characteristic of social health is social support, incorporating both the extent of a person's social networks and their perceived adequacy (Antonovsky, 1987).

Quality of life

Quality of life has been used by some researchers to encompass the broader notion of health and is also increasingly being used by researchers evaluating the effect of health care services. Quality of life includes an objective evaluation of life circumstances and a subjective evaluation of these circumstances. Fallowfield (1990) proposes four core domains in the quality of life:

- Psychological (e.g. depression)
- Social (e.g. engagement in social and leisure activities)
- Occupational (e.g. ability to carry out paid and/or domestic work)

■ Physical (e.g. pain, sleep, mobility).

Andrews and Withey (1976) have devised a non-verbal quality of life scale, the delighted–terrible faces (Figure 3.1).

Figure 3.1
Delighted–terrible faces: a non-verbal scale to assess self-ratings of quality of life and life satisfaction.
Here are some faces expressing various feelings. . . Which face comes closest to expressing how you feel about your health?

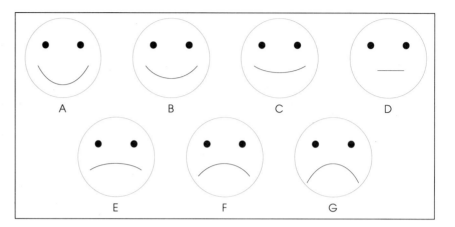

QALYs

The desire to include a measurement of health in evaluating health care outcomes has led to the development of quality-adjusted life years (QALYs). QALYs are an explicit attempt to include not just years of life saved but also the quality of life, when making resource allocation decisions regarding different medical procedures. The quality of life includes things such as freedom from pain and discomfort, and the ability to live independently. The assessment of quality of life is made by both health professionals and lay people. The QALY is the arithmetic product of life expectancy and an adjustment for the quality of the remaining life years gained (Balwin *et al.*, 1990). These two components are quite separate. QALYs are an important tool in making decisions about how to ration health care resources.

> **?**
>
> **These three people are all on the waiting list for a kidney transplant.**
>
> ■ Young mother of two
> ■ Unemployed single man of 50
> ■ Young married man with no children
> There is only one available donor kidney. Who would you recommend for the transplant and why?

There is much theoretical and methodological confusion in attempts to measure different aspects of positive health and a lack of consensus in how this may best be achieved. It is an area which is currently being refined and researched, and is undoubtedly important to any adequate conceptualization and measurement of health.

Conclusion

Measuring health is an important activity for health promoters, and is integral to the planning and evaluation of health promotion programmes. Yet there is no consensus on the best means to measure health, and a wide variety of methods have been used. Some are opportunistic, relying on data already collected and available such as the Jarman index and QALYs. The drawback of using these methods is that they use data which have been collected for specific reasons, often managerial or administrative. Other methods such as the Nottingham Profile have arisen from research which has addressed the issue of how to measure health. The fact that the concept 'health' can have so many different meanings, as outlined in Chapter 1, also contributes to the variety of different methods used. Some methods focus on one dimension of health, whereas others try to span different dimensions. It is also the case that different measures may suit different purposes. It is unlikely that any one method will ever prove to be a comprehensive measure of health, even if it combines different measurements within a weighted index. What is important then is to be specific about *why* you wish to measure health, and to then go on to select the most appropriate means of doing so, bearing in mind constraints on the time and money you have at your disposal.

> **?** **Match the measures of health with the health promoters.**
>
> *Health promoters*
> 1. Health visitor whose primary responsibility is for the health of mothers and under fives in a given area
> 2. Community development worker for a high-rise housing estate
> 3. Health promotion officer for a purchasing health authority
> 4. Environmental health officer
> 5. Community psychiatric nurse
>
> *Measures of health*
> - Pre-school children on the "at risk" social services register
> - Cases of food poisoning
> - Houses deemed to be unfit for human habitation
> - Registered drug addicts
> - Premature deaths from coronary heart disease
> - Joy riding and associated accidents
> - Patients on long-term medication for anxiety and depression
> - Take-up rates for childhood vaccinations.

Questions for further discussion

What are the advantages and disadvantages of measuring health as:

■ A negative variable (health is not being ill)
■ A positive variable (health is positive wellbeing)?

Thinking of your own work, how can you most usefully measure health?

Summary

This chapter has examined the reasons for attempting to measure health, and demonstrated that the most commonly used measures of health are in fact measures of ill health, disease and premature death. Recently there has been more activity directed towards trying to find ways of measuring health as an independent positive variable in its own right. Different approaches have been taken, ranging from measuring health as an objective property of people or environments, to measuring health as it is subjectively experienced and interpreted by people. These different approaches have been identified and described.

Further reading

Bowling A (1992) *Measuring Health*, Milton Keynes, Open University Press.

A useful summary of the different ways of measuring health.

Noack H (1991) "Conceptualizing and measuring health", in Badura B and Kickbusch I (eds) *Health Promotion Research: Towards a New Social Epidemiology* Copenhagen, World Health Organization Regional Office for Europe.

A useful article summarizing theoretical and practical issues concerning the measurement of health. Gives a framework for examining health.

Pickin C and St Leger S (1993)

Assessing Health Need Using the Life Cycle Framework, Buckingham, Open University Press.

A guide to using the life cycle framework to assess health needs. Includes useful sections on introduction to epidemiology and appendices on sources of data. Oriented towards the health services context.

References

Abberley P (1992) "A critique of the OPCS Disability Surveys", *Radical Statistics*, **51**, 7–21.

Andrews FM and Withey SB (1976) *Social Indicators of well-being: Americans' Perception of Life Quality*, New York, Plenum Press.

Antonovsky A (1987) *Unravelling the Mystery of Health: How People Manage Stress and Stay Well*, San Francisco, Jossey-Bass

Baldwin S, Godfrey C and Propper C (1990) *Quality of Life: Perspectives and Policies*, London, Routledge.

Bowling A (1992) *Measuring Health: A Review of Quality of Life Measurement Scales*, Milton Keynes, Open University Press.

Catford J (1983) "Positive health indicators – towards a new information base for health promotion", *Community Medicine*, **5**, 125–132

Chambers LW *et al.* (1982) "The McMaster health index questionnaire as a measure of quality of life for patients with rheumatoid disease", *Journal of Rheumatology*, **9**, 780–784.

Department of Epidemiology and Public Health Medicine, University of Bristol Medical School (1989) *Avon County Health Survey 1989: County Report.*

Department of Health (1992) *The Health of the Nation*, London, HMSO.

Dhooge Y and Dooris M (1988) *Working with Unemployment and Poverty: A Training Manual for Health Promotion*, London, South Bank Polytechnic.

Dupuy HJ (198) "The psychological general well-being (PGWB) index", in Wenger NK *et al.* (eds) *Assessment of quality of life in clinical trials of cardiovascular therapies*, pp 170–183, New York, Le Jacq.

Fallowfield L (1990) *The Quality of Life: The Missing Measurement in Health Care,* London, Souvenir Press.

Floud (1989) "Measuring European Inequality: The Use of Height Data", in Fox J (ed.) *Health Inequalities in European countries*, pp. 231–249, Aldershot, Gower.

Greenblatt HN (1975) *Measurement of Social Well-being in a General Population Survey,* Berkeley, Human Population Laboratory, California State Department of Health.

Hunt SM (1988) "Subjective health indicators and health promotion", *Health Promotion*, **3**, 3–34.

Hunt SM, McKenna SP and McEwan J *et al.* (1986) *Measuring Health Status*, London, Croom Helm.

Jarman B (1983) "Identification of underprivileged areas", *British Medical Journal*, **286**, 1705–1709.

McDowell I and Newell C (1987) *Measuring Health: A Guide to Rating Scales and Questionnaires*, New York, Oxford University Press.

Noack H (1991) "Conceptualizing and measuring health", in Badura B and Kickbusch I (eds) *Health Promotion Research: Towards a New Social Epidemiology*, pp. 85–112, Copenhagen, World Health Organisation Regional Office for Europe.

Oakley A and Oakley R (1981) "Sexism in official statistics", in Irvine J *et al.* (eds) *Demystifying Social Statistics*, pp. 172–189, London, Pluto Press.

Open University U205 Health and Disease Course Team (1985) *The Health of Nations: Book 3*, Milton Keynes, Open University.

Pickin C and St Leger S (1993) *Assessing Health Need Using the Life Cycle Framework*, Milton

Keynes, Open University Press.

Renne KS (1974) "Measurement of social health in a general population survey", *Social Sciences Research*, **3**, 25–44.

Roberts H (ed.) (1990) *Women's Health Counts*, London, Routledge.

Smyth M and Browne F (1992) *General Household Survey*, 1990 Series GHS No. 21, London, OPCS, HMSO.

Stewart AL *et al.* (1981) "Advances in the measurement of functional status: construction of aggregate indexes", *Medical Care*, **19**, 473–488.

Townsend P, Phillimore P and Beattie A (1987) *Health and Deprivation: Inequality and the North*, London, Croom Helm.

Townsend P, Davidson N and Whitehead M (1988) *Inequalities in Health: The Black Report and the Health Divide*, Harmondsworth, Penguin.

Wilkinson RG (1992) "Income distribution and life expectancy", *British Medical Journal*, **304**, 165–168.

World Health Organisation (1985) *Targets for Health for All*, Copenhagen, WHO Regional Office for Europe.

4 *The development of health education and health promotion*

Overview

Key points
- The different development of health education and health promotion
- Definitions of health education and health promotion, and the relationship between them
- The role of the World Health Organisation in health promotion

The process of attempting to promote health may include a whole range of interventions including:

- Those which foster healthy lifestyles
- Those which encourage access to services and involvement in health decisions
- Those which seek to promote an environment in which the healthy choice becomes the easier choice
- Those which educate about the body and keeping healthy.

Until the 1980s most of these interventions were referred to as "health education" and the practice was almost exclusively located within preventive medicine or, to a lesser extent, education. In recent years, the term health promotion has become widely used. This chapter considers whether this change in name signifies a difference in ideology, policy and practice. It discusses whether certain interventions are more concerned with health education or health promotion, or whether health promotion is a useful unifying concept which has brought together under one umbrella these different actions. Using a typology first suggested by Bunton and Macdonald (1992), it describes the development of health education and health promotion, and shows their interdependent development. The 19th century public health movement informed the health education of the earlier part of the 20th century which, in turn, informed the development of health promotion. It shows how the debate about the meaning of health education and health promotion has stemmed from a growing awareness that achieving "Health For All" requires not just changes in individual behaviour, but also, social and environmental change (Figure 4.1).

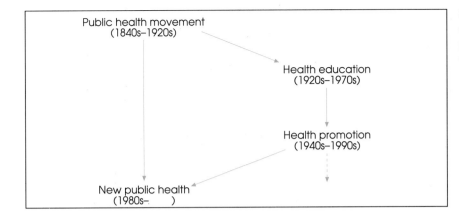

Figure 4.1 The development of health promotion (from Bunton and Macdonald, 1992).

The development of health education (see Table 4.1)

The origins of health education lie in the 19th century when epidemic disease eventually led to pressure for sanitary reform for the overcrowded industrial towns. Alongside the public health movement emerged the idea of educating the public for the good of its health. The Medical Officers of Health appointed to each town under the Public Health legislation of 1848 frequently disseminated everyday health advice on safeguards against "contagion". Voluntary associations were also formed including the London Statistical Society (1839), the Health of Towns Association (1842) and the Sanitary Institute (1876). The Temperance Movement held Band of Hope mass meetings, and through schools and churches lectured to young people on the virtue of abstinence. By the 1920s health education had become associated with diarrhoea, dirt, spitting and venereal disease! The evidence that between 10% and 20% of soldiers in the First World War had contracted venereal disease led to propaganda, one-off lectures and the first use of "shock–horror" techniques in which soldiers were shown lurid pictures of diseased genitals to dissuade them from having sex (Blythe, 1986).

- What do you consider to be the main features of health education?
- And what do you consider the main features of health promotion?
- Is your work mostly health education or health promotion?

 Health education slogans were produced in the 1920s by insurance companies keen to reduce health insurance claims:

- "Have a hot bath at least once a week"
- "Moderation in all things – every hour you steal from digestion will be reclaimed by indigestion"
- "Cultivate cheerfulness, hopefulness of mind and evenness of temper which are the most wonderful of remedial agencies"
- "Do not spit – it dries in the dust and other people breathe it in".

Changing patterns of morbidity and mortality shifted attention away from disease to personal behaviour. The Central Council for Health Education was established in 1927, paid for by local authority public health departments and public health doctors formed the majority of its membership. An extract from some of the tasks listed as important reflects an emphasis on information, and education to bring about change in personal habits and behaviour:

- The provision of better and cheaper posters and leaflets
- The provision of exhibits for exhibition
- The production of a readable monthly bulletin
- The provision of a panel of lecturers who really could lecture and hold an audience.

The Central Council was principally concerned with propaganda and instruction. During the Second World War it delivered 3799 lectures on sex education and venereal disease which were attended by 340 000 people (Amos, 1993).

The Health Education Council (HEC) which was set up in 1968 as a quango – a quasi non-governmental organization – reflected the Department of Health and Social Security's, as it then was, medical model of health. The members were drawn from public health, and the medical and dental professions with the inclusion of advertising and consumer affairs representatives. Its brief was to create a "climate of opinion generally favourable to health education, develop blanket programmes of education and selected priority subjects" (Cohen, 1964).

The HEC came to be associated with mass publicity campaigns including the employment of the advertising agency of Saatchi and Saatchi to design the "pregnant man" poster (Figure 4.2).

"Look after yourself" (LAY) was a major national programme launched in 1978. It articulated "the apparently simple notion that changes in ways of living, especially in youth and middle age, offer the prospect of large improvements in health and well-being. . ." (Health Education Council, 1978). Through public information and adult education classes in the community and the workplace, LAY was to act as a catalyst to encourage the uptake of healthy choices. The lead agency for health education consistently emphasized such mass campaigns and short-term initiatives. Sutherland, the first director of education and training at the Health Education Council, has vividly described the pressures and lobbying which led the HEC away from confrontation with vested interests, such as agriculture or tobacco, and kept it confined to mass-media campaigns despite evidence of their limited effect (Sutherland, 1987).

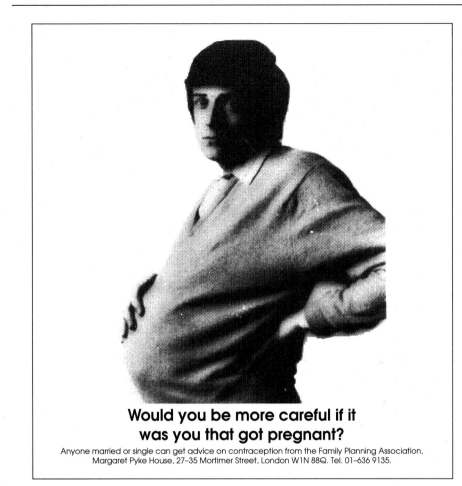

**Would you be more careful if it
was you that got pregnant?**

Anyone married or single can get advice on contraception from the Family Planning Association,
Margaret Pyke House, 27–35 Mortimer Street, London W1N 88Q. Tel. 01–636 9135.

Figure 4.2 The Health Education Authority's 'pregnant man' poster. © Saatchi & Saatchi.

Table 4.1 The development of health education in the 20th century

1900	Concern for infant and child health: health visitors, mother and baby clinics, school medical service (1908)
1906–1914	Liberal Government reforms including: national insurance and old age pensions
1919	Ministry of Health. Numerous voluntary organisations producing leaflets and posters including National Association for the Prevention of Tuberculosis, Health and Cleanliness Council, British Red Cross
1927	Central Council for Health Education of medical officers of health, local authority associations and health insurance committees
1940–1945	Major campaigns e.g. to promote diphtheria immunization. Rates rose from 8% to 62%. Emphasis on venereal disease education.
1946	Responsibility for health education transferred to Ministry of Health from local authorities
1948	National Health Service
1957	First course of training for health education specialists at London University Institute of Education. First Health Education Officers employed by local authorities

1964	Cohen Committee to consider the future of health education recommended a strong central body
1968	Health Education Council set up, funded and appointed by the newly established Department of Health and Social Security (DHSS)
1970s	High profile mass-media campaigns on smoking, immunization, family planning. Employment of Saatchi and Saatchi advertising agency. Support for curriculum development work in schools. Support for training and research
1974	NHS reorganization: regional, area and district health authorities, consensus maangement by muiltidisciplinary District Management Team. Creation of Community Health Councils.
1976	*Prevention and Health: Everybody's Business* published by DHSS followed by numerous reports on prevention
1977	World Health Organisation declaration at Alma Ata committing members to the principles of Health For All 2000
1982	Reorganization of the NHS to offer more local community structure: district health authorities. Publication of the Black Report on inequalities in health
1984	Griffiths Report recommended general managers for the NHS, reducing health professionals' role in management
1986	World Health Organisation Ottawa Charter
1987	White Paper *Promoting Better Health*. Culmination of reports on primary health care and neighbourhood nursing (Cumberledge Report). Family doctors to be encouraged to carry out health promotion linked to financial incentives for health checks and reaching targeted vaccination levels.
	Health Education Council disbanded. Health Education Authority established as a special health authority within the NHS in England. The Health Promotion Authority for Wales and the Health Education Board (1991, renamed) in Scotland are set up.
	Ministerial groups focus on the issues of HIV/AIDS and drug misuse. These issues receive relatively large sums of money. Major advertising including the first AIDS awareness campaign "Don't die of ignorance".
	"Look after your heart" major campaign to raise awareness of coronary heart disease
1988	Acheson Report on public health in England
1990	NHS and Community Care Act divided the NHS into purchaser and provider units. The purchasing authority has responsibility for determining health needs and commissioning services from provider units
1992	*The Health of the Nation* strategy published. Identifies five key target areas:
	coronary heart disease; accidents; mental health; sexual health; cancers

By the 1970s there was an increasing recognition that health policy could not continue to be confined to clinical and medical services, which were proving both expensive and not improving the health status of the population. Health education and the prevention of disease represented a means of cutting costs and an ideology which could place the onus of responsibility with the individual.

The Government document *Prevention and Health: Everybody's Business* (DHSS, 1976) was published in 1976 and encapsulates a behavioural approach which sees health problems as the result of individual lifestyles.

> "To a large extent though, it is clear that the weight of responsibility for his own health lies on the shoulders of the individual himself. The smoking-related diseases, alcoholism and other drug dependencies, obesity and its consequences, and the sexually transmitted diseases are among the preventable problems of our time and, in relation to all of these, the individual must decide for himself" (DHSS, 1976).

The message of the document is that improving health depends on individuals changing the way they live in order to avoid "lifestyle" diseases. A decade later in 1987 a similar message was put forward by the White Paper *Promoting Better Health* which suggested that the major killer diseases could be avoided if people took greater responsibility for their own health (Department of Health, 1987). Smith (1991) has argued that "The Health of the Nation" strategy is also permeated by a philosophy of individualism despite the acknowledgement in the strategy that "responsibilities for action are similarly widely spread from individuals to government" (Department of Health, 1992).

Health education as prevention

In Chapter 1 we saw that there are many different meanings attached to the concept of health but the notion of health being "the absence of disease or infirmity" is a dominant one. Different perceptions about the nature of health underpin the nature of health education. Although some definitions of health education suggest it may be concerned with the enhancement of health as well as the prevention of ill health, in practice the dominance of the medical model has frequently meant it has had a negative focus. Health education has been aimed at preventing specific diseases, often through targeting high-risk groups who have an increased likelihood of developing that disease. Health education then is seen as disease prevention and interventions are designed to prevent ill health. Thus health education is often categorized as concerned with primary, secondary or tertiary prevention.

Primary prevention seeks to avoid the onset of ill health by the detection of high-risk groups and the provision of advice and counselling. Examples of primary prevention would include immunization and cervical cytology. Secondary prevention seeks to shorten episodes of illness and prevent the progression of ill health through early diagnosis and treatment. Examples include education about medication, advice on healthy eating for a diabetic, relaxation for cardiac patients. Tertiary prevention seeks to limit disability or complications arising from an irreversible condition. Examples include education about the use of a disability aid and rehabilitation.

? The *Health of the Nation* strategy identifies mental illness as one of five key target areas. It outlines the following measures.

1. Primary prevention to include:
- Redundancy and retirement counselling
- Genetic screening and advice on the avoidance of drugs in pregnancy
- Befriending schemes for young mothers
- Early detection and management of emotional and physical child abuse
- Increasing the individual's ability to recognize stress and look after themselves.

2. Secondary prevention to include:
- Early detection and management of depression in primary care
- Developing personal coping strategies to minimize the effects of conditions, for example, hearing voices.

3. Tertiary prevention to include:
- Countering discrimination in health provision to people with a history of mental illness
- Developing coping strategies for carers
- Providing respite care for people with chronic mental illness.

Do you consider these measures to be promoting mental health or preventing mental illness? What other measures might you include in a positive mental health strategy?

Towards a definition of health education

Through this brief history of health education, we can see how both medicine and education have informed its development. The rationale of health education has been to inform people about the prevention of disease and to motivate them to change their behaviour, through persuasion and mass communication techniques, and to equip them through education with the skills for a healthy lifestyle. For some health educators, this means providing people with information about health and disease issues. *The Health of the Nation* (Department of Health, 1992) strategy defines the aim of health education as being "to ensure that individuals are able to exercise informed choice when selecting the lifestyle which they adopt". Others may go further and suggest that health education also involves persuading people to adopt healthy behaviours. What does count as health education and what criteria would you use to decide?

?   **Consider these two definitions of health education. What features distinguish health education according to these two authors?**

- "Health education is any planned activity which promotes health or illness related learning, that is, some relatively permanent change in an individual's competence or disposition" (Tones, 1990)
- "Health education is not about behavioural change, and it is not about overt political action to affect the determinants of health. Rather health education is about enabling – supporting people to set their own health agendas, agendas they can then implement in ways decided by themselves collectively or as individuals" (French, 1990).

These two definitions contained in an issue of the *Health Education Journal* which, for over a decade, has carried on the debate about the concepts of health education and health promotion, make clear that health education has two distinct elements: it is planned and it involves a voluntary change. However, whilst Tones clearly states that health education is aimed to bring about a change in attitude or skills, French suggests overt behavioural change is not its intention.

One of the paradoxes of health education and a prevailing professional dilemma is the question of voluntarism or free choice. On the one hand health education is based on an authority model derived from both medicine and education. It is the health educator or doctor who decides if there is a health need and the adequacy of an individual's lifestyle, who decides the nature of the intervention and the most effective means of communication, who tries to ensure compliance, and who will decide if the intervention has "worked". When we look at the practice of health education, we might be led to believe that health education is the *giving* of information. However, for many health educators education is a means of *drawing out*. Clients are not "empty vessels" who will rationally change their behaviour once provided with the relevant information, advice or guidance. They seek neither to coerce nor to persuade, both because this is unlikely to be effective but also because it is unethical. The health educator is a facilitator and enabler rather than an expert. Rather than telling a client what to do, the health educator works with the client to identify their needs and work towards an informed choice, even when this may lead to health-damaging behaviour.

 How should health promoters work with pregnant women who smoke?

- Health Promoter A tells her clients to stop smoking for the sake of the unborn child and gives her clients information illustrating the risks to the foetus.
- Health promoter B talks with her clients about their reasons for smoking and the most important times when they smoke. She then works out a programme with her client to cut down on less necessary cigarettes, working towards giving up.

Which approach comes closest to your own preferred way of working?

These two strands of voluntarism and authoritarianism reflect the historical development of health education, as educationists and social scientists challenged the mainstream of preventive medicine contesting the assumption that health education could, or indeed should, seek to bring about behaviour change through information or persuasion. Thus emerged the principle of self-empowerment which many argue is central to the practice of health education (Tones, 1992). Empowerment is an approach which enables people to take charge of their lives including changing their behaviour if they so wish. The range of approaches to health education are outlined and discussed in the following chapter. They range from the medical model, focusing on health surveillance and achieving behaviour change, to the educational model which relies on the exploration of attitudes and values. Alongside these are the approaches more closely aligned to health promotion, such as community development, which emphasizes the need to take collective action for health, and a political model which focuses on the need to influence decision makers at local and national level.

? Consider these descriptions of the work of a nurse on an acute medical ward and a health promotion officer working with young people. Would you consider them to be practising health education or health promotion? What criteria do you use to make your judgement?

- "Patient education for coronary care is carried out one to one with information booklets. The overall aim is to alleviate anxiety, promote recovery and educate about the cause of the attack to get the patient back to normal and even healthier. Patients may be given factual information about the working of the heart, be taught relaxation exercises, encouraged to talk about concerns such as sex after a heart attack. They will be educated about their medication, how to eat healthily keeping their weight down and curbing their cholesterol intake, and ways to increase physical activity."

> **(cont.)**
> ■ "Health education in schools passes on knowledge, allows for discussion and leads to understanding. It gives young people the freedom to choose and make health decisions and at the same time it asserts an appreciation and respect for the choices of others. The end result should lead to positive pleasure for the young person whilst enabling them to remain healthy and disease-free."
>
> A key difference between these two interventions is their aims. In the coronary care unit, the nurse is actively engaged in disease prevention – to prevent a further heart attack. In the school, the Health Promotion Officer aims to equip young people with the information and skills for a healthy lifestyle. In both cases, the health promoter aims for behaviour change, more obviously so in the coronary care unit. Both use similar educational methods of providing information, encouraging clients to reflect on their attitudes and experience, and providing opportunities to practise skills.

The public health movement

When we try to characterize current practice in health promotion, we must look for its influences in health education but also in the public health movement. The overcrowded, insanitary conditions in 19th century industrial towns led to pressure for reforms to promote the public health. Edwin Chadwick, who administered the Poor Law, reported in 1842 on "the sanitary condition of the labouring population" that the ill health experienced by the poor was largely the result of poor sanitation and hygiene at home and at work.

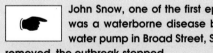 John Snow, one of the first epidemiologists, discovered that cholera was a waterborne disease by tracing an outbreak in 1854 to one water pump in Broad Street, Soho. When the handle of the pump was removed, the outbreak stopped.

By 1875 a Public Health Act made provision for the control of the water supply, sewage disposal and animal slaughter. At the turn of the century, the Boer War exposed a crisis of fitness in the nation. A total of 40% of army recruits were rejected on health grounds. The period before the First World War thus saw a spate of Government welfare reforms including school meals, the school medical service and National Insurance.

Many of the 19th century social reformers attributed the behaviour of the poor to their social conditions (see Figure 4.3). Crime, unrest and "moral depravity" were seen as having their roots in overcrowding and squalor. But the public health movement owed little to the benevolence of the middle classes towards the

Figure 4.3 A portion of Snow's map of the spread of cholera in Soho. Blue bars represent the number of fatal cases in each house. The position of the Broad Street pump from which all the victims had obtained water is also marked.

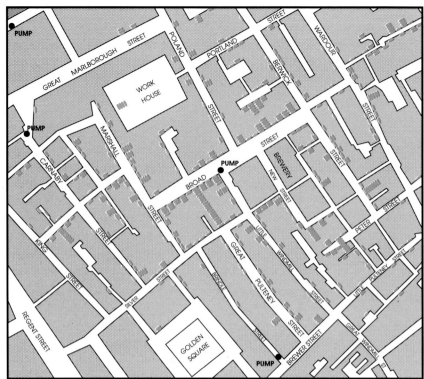

poor, and much to an awareness that a competitive work and fighting force to match the strong nations of Europe would need an improvement in the health of the nation. (Wohl, 1983) Rapid industrialization also posed a threat to social stability and the mid-19th century saw several measures to maintain public order and limit the size of public gatherings. By the late 19th century, as the fear of disease receded, the initiative of public health moved away from municipal reform and a focus on the environment to biomedical aspects of illness, which later resulted in the lifestyle approach to public health and to comprehensive immunization and screening programmes led by the Medical Officers of Health.

Reasons of economy, competitiveness, prevention of radical movements – these were all influences on 19th-century health promotion.

■ Are the same arguments used today?
■ How is health promotion justified in the late 20th century?

" The most pestilential of these places, when once put in a wholesome condition, could be maintained in that state at a comparatively small expense; . . . it follows, that the prevention of evil, rather than the mitigation of the consequences of it, is not only the most beneficent but the most economical course" (Southwood Smith, Appendix C2 to Fifth Report to the Poor Law Commission, 1839).

Throughout the 20th century there have also been examples of legislation which have had a profound effect on public health. The British people, for example, are said to have been at their healthiest during the Second World War when emergency food rationing limited their sugar and fat intake, and increased reliance on home grown cereals and vegetables.

The new public health

In 1988 a commission of inquiry reported on public health in England. Known as the Acheson report after its chairman, Sir Donald Acheson, then Chief Medical Officer at the Department of Health, it defined public health as "the science and art of preventing disease, prolonging life and promoting health through the organized efforts of society". The report recommended a new post to replace the old District Medical Officer – a Director of Public Health. It is, however, local authorities and not the health service who have been most active in their support for public health and have supported the use of legislation to produce a more health-promoting environment. Regulations, fiscal measures, policies and voluntary codes of practice may all be used to provide the population with the opportunities to make the healthier choice the easier choice. This might mean working towards no smoking in the workplace, the production of leaner meat, the introduction of alcohol labelling and warnings. What has been called the "new public health" also means statutory and voluntary agencies working together to assess the implications for health in all public policies – agriculture, energy, transport, defence, economic development, employment, housing, education and leisure.

Consider the following newspaper headlines. Is there a need for a new public health?

- Thousands of chickens slaughtered in salmonella scare
- Hamburgers banned in schools in case of mad cow disease
- 10% of London children living in temporary accommodation
- Outrage at closure of coal mines
- 6000 people killed each year in road traffic accidents
- Three million unemployed and rising
- Surfers protest at sewage dumping
- Chips, chips and more chips – the school dinner of the nineties.

? **Milio's pioneering work in Canada and North America (1986) has analysed the effect on health of various public sectors and shown how alternative policy decisions could enhance health.**

- Can you think of examples for a healthy public energy policy?
- Or transport?
- Or agriculture?

Public health measures often involve confrontation with powerful vested interests. The most obvious example is the reluctance of successive Governments to ban tobacco advertising despite strong evidence that a ban on advertising does reduce the numbers of new smokers. Hunt (1989) draws our attention to the implications of private car ownership for the public health. She claims this has escaped serious attention because most people with influence have a lifestyle in which the car plays a prominent role; enormous amounts of revenue are raised from taxes on petrol and the new car industry is a major UK employer. Thus she claims, "attention is diverted from the enormous impact of car use on disease, death, disability, quality of life, the integrity of the environment, social intercourse, social inequalities and the huge financial cost to the public purse".

> **?**
>
> McKinlay (1979), in persuading us of the need to refocus upstream, tells a story:
> "There I am standing by the shore of a swiftly flowing river and I hear the cry of a drowning man. So I jump into the river, put my arms around him, pull him to shore and apply artifical respiration. Just when he begins to breathe, there is another cry for help. So I jump into the river, reach him, pull him to shore, apply artificial respiration, and then just as he begins to breathe, another cry for help. So back in the river again, without end, goes the sequence. You know I am so busy jumping in, pulling them to shore, applying artificial respiration, that I have no time to see who the hell is upstream pushing them all in".
>
> The concept of refocusing upstream is a powerful and persuasive argument for health promotion. It can help us to reorientate our thinking from a belief that medical care can, or will, solve most health problems towards prevention. You might like to discuss these fundamental questions with colleagues:
>
> ■ What examples can you think of in your own work of short-term problem-specific tinkering?
> ■ What would a reorientation upstream involve?
> ■ Who do you think is pushing people in?

The development of health promotion and the contribution of the World Health Organisation (WHO)

Health promotion is a term that has been widely used in the last 10 years but in many different ways. The term "health promotion" was first used in 1974 by the Canadian Minister of National Health and Welfare, Marc Lalonde. *A New Perspective on the Health of Canadians* argued that the major causes of death and disease lay not in biomedical characteristics but in the environment and in individual behaviours and lifestyles. In the following decades, the World Health Organisation was to build on this and play a key part in shifting the emphasis from medical care to primary *health* care.

In 1977 the World Health Assembly at Alma Ata committed all member countries to the principles of *Health For All 2000* (HFA 2000) that there "should be the attainment by all the people of the world by the year 2000 of a level of health that will permit them to lead a socially and economically productive life." The WHO made explicit five key principles for health promotion:

1. It involves the population as a whole in the context of their everyday life, rather than focusing on people at risk for specific diseases.
2. It is directed towards action on the causes or determinants of health to ensure that the total environment which is beyond the control of individuals is conducive to health.
3. It combines diverse, but complementary, methods or approaches including communication, education, legislation, fiscal measures, organizational change, community development and spontaneous local activities against health hazards.
4. It aims particularly at effective public participation supporting the principle of self-help movements and encouraging people to find their own ways of managing the health of their community.
5. While health promotion is basically an activity in the health and social fields and not a medical service, health professionals – particularly in primary health care – have an important role in nurturing and enabling health promotion.

The context for the development of broad-based health strategies will thus need to be based on equity, community participation and intersectoral collaboration. The WHO also identify that improvements in lifestyles, environmental conditions and health care will have little effect if certain fundamental conditions are not met. These include:

■ Peace and freedom from the fear of war
■ Equal opportunity for all and social justice
■ Satisfaction of basic needs
■ Political commitment and public support (WHO, 1985).

The WHO launched a programme for health promotion in 1984, and conferences at Ottawa (1986), Adelaide (1988) and Sandsvall (1991) have further outlined areas for action. The principles of health promotion are developed in the Ottawa Charter which outlines these areas as important for health promotion:

1. Building a healthy public policy
2. Creating supportive environments
3. Developing personal skills
4. Strengthening community action
5. Reorienting health services.

It also included three ways in which health could be promoted:

■ **Advocacy.** Evidence on individual and community health needs should be collected showing the implications for health of social and political issues. People's knowledge and understanding of the factors which affect health should be increased and health promoters should work to empower people so they may argue their own right to health and negotiate changes in their personal environment.

■ **Enablement**. Health promotion should aim to reduce differences in current health status and ensure equal opportunities to enable all people to achieve their full health potential. Health promoters should work to increase knowledge and understanding, and individual coping strategies. In an attempt to improve access to health, health promoters should work with individuals and communities to identify needs and help to develop support networks in the neighbourhood.

■ **Mediation.** Health promotion requires coordination and cooperation by many agencies and sectors. Health promoters have a major role to mediate between different interests by providing evidence and advice to local groups; by influencing local and national policy through lobbying, media campaigns and participation in working groups.

In these declarations by the WHO we can see how the emphasis has moved away from prevention of specific diseases or the detection of risk groups towards the health and well-being of whole populations. Instead of experts and professionals diagnosing problems, the people themselves define health issues of relevance to them in their local community. Teachers, primary health-care workers, workplace managers, social and welfare workers can all be involved in promoting health. Instead of health being seen as the responsibility of individuals alone, the social factors determining health are taken into account, and health is viewed as a collective responsibility of society.

Health education and health promotion – is there a difference?

"Health Promotion has come to represent a unifying concept for those who recognize the need for change in the ways and conditions of living in order to promote health. Health promotion represents a mediating strategy between people and their environments, synthesizing personal choice and social responsibility in health to create a healthier future" (WHO, 1984).

The WHO does distinguish between health promotion and prevention; health education is seen as an integral part of health promotion in conjunction with the field of prevention. For many health promoters, however, the debate about the difference has been more a move to redefine professional boundaries, and to revitalize a tired and underfunded service than a shift in ways of thinking (Rawson, 1988). Specialist workers who were previously known as Health Education Officers have frequently changed their title to Health Promotion Officers and lately, to Health Promotion Specialists without necessarily changing their professional role. Many professions, including nurses, have found health promotion part of an expanding job description. The list of competencies for a first level nurse includes "to promote the health of clients" and a major part of the new nursing curriculum of Project 2000 is devoted to health promotion. These developments reflect the arguments presented in this book, that it is health not illness or disease which should underpin health care work.

Health promotion has become what Galli (1978) calls an "essentially contested concept". It is used differently by different people. For example, the way the Government uses the term "health promotion" when they refer to screening clinics in primary health care is very different from the holistic and political concept of the World Health Organisation. Even more confusingly, some people have used the term health promotion to describe those aspects of health education which involve high-profile publicity events and emulate commercial marketing techniques, what Williams (1984) calls "slick salesmanship".

It has been claimed that the term health promotion has been so widely used and been given so many meanings that it risks becoming meaningless (Tannahill,1985). One solution to this confusion of meanings is to use "health promotion" as an umbrella term to cover all interventions that promote health, including health education.

> "Health promotion incorporates all measures deliberately designed to promote health and handle disease. . . A major feature of health promotion is undoubtedly the importance of 'healthy public policy' with its potential for achieving social change via legislation, fiscal, economic and other forms of 'environmental engineering'." (Tones, 1990).

Using a phrase first coined by Milio (1986) and which has come to encapsulate health promotion – "making the healthier choice the easier choice" – Draper and colleagues make a sharp distinction between health promotion and health education, but clearly saw the latter as part of a broader process.

> "The terms health promotion and health education are not interchangeable. Health promotion covers all aspects of those activities which seek to improve the health status of individuals and communities. It therefore includes both health education and all attempts to produce environmental and legislative change conducive to good health. Put another way, health promotion is concerned with making healthier choices easier choices" (Dennis et al., 1982).

Tannahill expands on an earlier model for defining and planning health promotion and makes a distinction between health education, prevention and what he describes as health protection (Downie *et al.*, 1990). Health protection involves public and fiscal policies aimed at preventing ill health, and promoting better health such as the wearing of seat belts. Tannahill sees health promotion as an umbrella for equally important related activities but not as a unique activity itself.

It is clear from these quotations that a key feature which distinguishes health promotion from health education is that it involves environmental and political action. Health education is distinguished by the centrality accorded to autonomy and voluntarism. The underlying principles of health education include the promotion of self-esteem and non-coercion (French, 1990). Whilst health educators may respect cultural norms and take account of the social and economic constraints which affect people's ability to make health choices, essentially people are facilitated to make their own informed choice about health behaviour. For those who believe that the roots of ill health lie in the social structure, this emphasis on choice is merely illusory. In Chapter 6 we shall explore further the limits to freedom of choice and how far an ethical principle such as the promotion of autonomy can govern our practice as health educators and health promoters. Conversely, adherents of health education might describe health promotion measures, such as legislation for the compulsory wearing of safety belts or smoking restrictions in public places, or the fluoridation of the water supply as "social engineering". Such activities, by limiting individual choice, might be deemed unethical or undesirable.

In practice, health education and health promotion have come to reflect different political orientations which can be characterized as the individual versus structural approaches. What happens when the two concepts are polarized is that health education comes to be seen as a narrow field of activity which seeks to explain health status by reference to individual lifestyles and is a process largely determined by an expert. In its emphasis on personal responsibility, it sees a minimal role for the state and, thus, has come to be associated with a conservative viewpoint. Health promotion, because it sees health and wealth as inextricably linked, and seeks to address the root causes of ill health and problems of inequity, is seen as radical and challenging.

It is not helpful to debate whether one form of activity is better or worse than the other: both are necessary. Health promotion may involve lobbying and political advocacy, but it may just as easily involve working with individuals and groups to enhance their knowledge and understanding of the factors affecting their health. In practice, health education and health promotion interact and overlap with each other. The process of identifying the different values which underpin different models of health promotion is discussed further in Chapter 5.

Conclusion

This chapter, by tracing the historical development, has shown that it is possible to distinguish between disease prevention, health education and health promotion. We take the view that health education is different in aim and method from health promotion but is very much part of that wider process of building a healthy public policy and getting that policy accepted.

Many health workers are strongly committed to health education and the promotion of health. However, this has often been manifested in one-to-one programmes limited to providing information. Many may be daunted by the broad definition of health promotion and feel that this broad approach is beyond their professional remit. Indeed, it would not be possible for any one worker or group to bring about the changes needed for a health-promoting society. It is important that we remind ourselves of the WHO view which describes the process of promoting health as not only involving political change, but also enabling people to take more control over their own health and equipping them with the means for well-being. Health promotion thus includes increasing individual knowledge about the functions of the body and ways of preventing illness, raising competence in using the health care system, and raising awareness about the political and environmental factors that influence health. The process, which includes individual, group and community change, and incorporates a range of strategies, is shown diagrammatically in Figure 4.4.

"The new methods of health promotion are introducing new forms of social regulation which are not ostensibly oppressive or obviously controlling. In these, often innocuous-looking forms, they nevertheless enter and regulate our lives in new ways and bring with them new concerns for our civil liberties and rights" (Bunton, 1992).

Think of some examples of social regulation aimed to promote health. Do you share this concern at the extension of health promotion into areas beyond "health"?

Questions for further discussion

■ Is it useful to try to distinguish between health education and health promotion? Which term would you choose to describe your work in improving people's health?
■ How do you explain the emphasis on health promotion in contemporary health care work?

Summary

This chapter has looked at the origins of the practice of health education and health promotion. It has shown the importance of the public health movement in promoting health and the influence

Figure 4.4 The process of health promotion

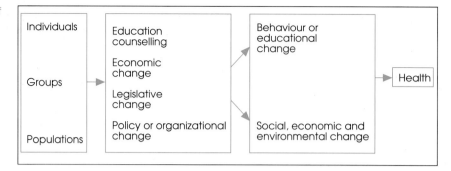

> ### ? The following activities have all been undertaken by health promoters. Which types of activity would you consider to be part of your work?
>
> - Running an exercise group for elderly people in a day centre
> - Immunizing a child
> - Lobbying your employer to provide showers in the workplace to encourage people to cycle or take exercise at lunchtime
> - Running a stress-management group at work
> - Drawing up a healthy eating programme for a diabetic
> - Working with a GP practice to monitor prescription of benzodiazepine
> - Putting up a display for National No Smoking Day
> - Researching the needs of alcohol users
> - Planning an individual care plan for a young cerebral palsy patient
> - Offering advice to the purchaser of HIV services in the Health Authority
> - Organizing a parent education class at a local school
> - Setting up a stall in the local market to offer health information
> - Facilitating a women's health group
> - Offering advice on social and financial supports available to clients
> - Organizing a cooking group for 'people living with AIDS' in the community
> - Carrying out hearing tests in a local school
>
> Look again at your responses. You will notice that some of these activities relate more closely to health education and some to health promotion. At the start of this chapter, you were asked how your work illustrates the difference between health education and health promotion. Have your views changed?

of the World Health Organisation in shifting perceptions about the prevention of disease to the enhancement of health and well-being. It has explored some of the definitions of health education and health promotion, and set the boundaries for these processes, concluding that health education is an important part of the wider process of health promotion.

Further reading

Ashton J and Seymour H (1988) *The New Public Health*, Milton Keynes, Open University Press.

A readable account of the historical development of public health that, using Liverpool as an example shows how, in the New Public Health, the health implications of public policy are addressed.

Beattie A *et al.* (eds) (1993) *Health and Wellbeing: A Reader*, Milton Keynes, Open University Press.

An excellent collection of articles to accompany the Open University course K258 "Health and Wellbeing". The reader illustrates competing perspectives on health in wider debates about social planning and policy making.

Bunton R and Macdonald G (1992) *Health Promotion: Disciplines and Diversity*, London, Routledge.

An interesting collection of contributions which traces the theoretical roots of health promotion through the disciplines of psychology, sociology, education and epidemiology.

Downie RS, Fyfe C and Tannahill A (1990) *Health Promotion; Models and Values*, Oxford, Oxford Medical Publications.

A useful introduction which outlines the debate about boundaries for health promotion

Health Education Journal

Editions from 1984 have carried the debate about the difference between health education and health promotion. In particular: 1984 (43, nos 2 and 3); 1985, (44, nos 2 and 4); 1986, (45, no. 2); 1990, (49, no. 1).

References

Acheson D (1988) *Public Health in England*, Report of the Committee of Inquiry into the future development of the Public Health Function, London, HMSO.

Amos A (1993) "In her own best interests: women and health education, a review of the last 50 years", *Health Education Journal*, **52**, 3.

Beattie A (1991) "Knowledge and control in health promotion: a test case for social policy and social theory", in Gabe J, Calnan M and Bury M (eds) *The Sociology of the Health Service*, London, Routledge.

Blythe M (1986) "A century of health education", *Health and Hygiene*, **7**, 105–115.

Bunton R (1992) "More than a woolly jumper: health promotion as social regulation" *Critical Public Health*, **3**, 4–11.

Bunton R and Macdonald G (1992) *Health Promotion: Disciplines and Diversity*, London, Routledge.

Chadwick E (1842) *Report on the Sanitary Condition of the Labouring Population of England*, London, HMSO.

Cohen Committee (1964) *Health Education*, Report of a Joint Committee of the Central and Scottish Health Services Councils, London, HMSO.

Dennis J *et al.* (1982) "Health promotion in the re-organised NHS" *The Health Services*, 26/11/82.

Department of Health (1987) *Promoting Better Health*, London, HMSO.

Department of Health (1992) *The Health of the Nation*, London, HMSO.

Department of Health and Social Security (1976) *Prevention and Health; Everybody's Business*, London, HMSO.

French J (1990) "Boundaries and horizons, the role of health education within health promotion", *Health Education Journal*, **49**, 7–10.

Downie RS, Fyfe C and Tannahill A (1990) *Health Promotion: Models and Values*, Oxford, Oxford Medical Publications.

Galli N (1978) *Foundations and Principles of Health Education*, Chichester, Wiley.

Health Education Council (1978) *Annual Report*, London, HEC.

Hunt SM (1989) "The public health implications of private cars" in Martin C and McQueen D (eds) *Readings for a New Public Health*, Edinburgh, Edinburgh University Press.

McKinlay JB (1979) "A case for refocussing upstream: the political economy of health" in Jaco EG (ed.) *Patients, Physicians and Illness*, Basingstoke, Macmillan.

Milio N (1986) *Promoting Health Through Public Policy*, Ottawa, Canadian Public Health Association.

Rawson D and Grigg C (1988) *Purpose and Practice in Health Education*, London, South Bank Polytechnic/HEA.

Smith R (1991) "First steps towards a strategy for health", *British Medical Journal*, **303**, 297–299.

Sutherland I (1987) *Health Education: Half a Policy*, Cambridge, National Extension College.

Tannahill A (1985) "What is health promotion?", *Health Education Journal*, **44**, 4.

Tones K (1990) "Why theorise: ideology in health education", *Health Education Journal* , **49**, 1.

Tones K (1992) Empowerment and the promotion of health" *Journal of the Institute of Health Education*, **30**, 4.

Williams G (1984) "Health promotion – caring concern or slick salesmanship", *Journal of Medical Ethics*, **10**.

Wohl AS (1983) *Endangered Lives: Public Health in Victorian Britain*, London, Dent & Sons.

World Health Organisation (1984) *Health Promotion: A Discussion Document on Concepts and Principles*, Geneva, WHO.

World Health Organisation (1985) *Targets for Health for All*, Geneva, WHO.

Models and approaches to health promotion

5

Overview

The diversity in concepts of health, influences on health and ways of measuring health leads, not surprisingly, to a number of different approaches to health promotion. The previous chapter began to explore the concepts of health education and health promotion. In this chapter, five different approaches will be discussed:

■ Medical or preventive
■ Behaviour change
■ Educational
■ Empowerment
■ Social change.

These approaches will be examined in terms of their different aims, methods and means of evaluation.

It is likely that one of these approaches will be more familiar to you from your work. For example, teachers are likely to identify most with the educational approach, whereas nurses might feel most comfortable with the medical approach. By examining different stances towards carrying out health promotion, you will be able to consider your own approach critically. It may be that there are aspects you would like to incorporate into your work and you may wish to adopt different elements from the different approaches.

Identifying the different approaches is primarily a descriptive process. Alongside these descriptions is emerging a theoretical framework for health promotion which provides a representation in the form of models. The last part of this chapter is an outline of the principal theoretical models of health promotion and a discussion of their usefulness in explaining health promotion practice.

Key points
■ Different approaches to health promotion:
  ■ Medical
  ■ Behaviour change
  ■ Educational
  ■ Empowerment
  ■ Social change
■ Aspects of these approaches:
  ■ Aims
  ■ Methods
  ■ Means of evaluation
■ The importance of theory in health promotion
■ Different models of health promotion

The medical approach

Aims

This approach focuses on activity which aims to reduce morbidity and premature mortality. Activity is targeted towards whole populations or high-risk groups. This kind of health promotion seeks to increase medical interventions which will prevent ill health and premature death, such as immunization and screening.

The medical approach to health promotion is popular because:

1. It has high status because it uses scientific methods, such as epidemiology (the study of the pattern of diseases in society).
2. In the short term, prevention and the early detection of disease is much cheaper than treatment and care of people who have become ill. Of course, in the long term, this may not be the case as people live longer and experience degenerative conditions and draw pensions for a longer period.
3. It is an expert-led, or top-down, type of intervention. This kind of activity reinforces the authority of medical professionals who are recognized as having the expert knowledge needed to achieve the desired results.
4. There have been spectacular successes in public health as a result of using this approach, for example, the worldwide eradication of smallpox as a result of the vaccination programme.

As we have seen in Chapter 1, the medical approach is conceptualized around the absence of disease. It does not seek to promote positive health and can be criticized for ignoring the social and environmental dimensions of health. In addition, the medical approach encourages dependency on medical knowledge and removes health decisions from the people concerned. Thus, health care workers are encouraged to persuade patients to co-operate and comply with treatment.

Public health medicine is the branch of medicine which specializes in prevention, and most day to day preventive work is carried out by the community health services which include health visitors and district nurses. Health promotion has recently been prioritized within the primary-care setting. This will tend to reinforce certain aspects of health promotion (those which are funded, such as the collection of health status statistics) at the expense of others (such as the facilitation of post-natal support groups). The medical approach reinforces not just the medicalization of life but also the medical hierarchy, where doctors have authority over other health care workers.

Methods

The principle of preventive services such as immunization and screening is that they are targeted to groups at risk from a particular condition. Whilst immunization requires a certain level of take-up for it to be effective, screening is offered to specific groups. For example, cervical screening every 3 years is offered to sexually active women over 20.

For screening to be effective for the condition or disease:

■ It should have a long preclinical phase so that a screening test will not miss its signs
■ Earlier treatment should improve the outcomes
■ The test should be sensitive, i.e. it should detect all those with the disease
■ The test should be specific, i.e. it should detect *only* those with the disease
■ The test should be acceptable, easy to perform and safe
■ It should be cost effective, i.e. the number of tests performed should yield a number of positive cases.

> **?** **Consider the example of amniocentesis – the testing of the amniotic fluid around a foetus to detect chromosomal abnormalities. Does this test meet the criteria for effective screening outlined above?**
>
> In most districts, amniocentesis is only offered to women over the age of 37 and those with a family history of chromosomal abnormality. Yet 90% of children with Down's syndrome are born to mothers under 37 simply because more women in this age group have babies. Amniocentesis is not a simple test. It carries a risk of miscarriage. It can also only be performed after 14–16 weeks of pregnancy when a possible termination is more difficult. It is less than 100% sensitive and therefore some women may go away falsely reassured. A termination and/or counselling is the only intervention available.

Preventive procedures need to be based on a sound rationale derived from epidemiological evidence. The medical approach also relies on having an infrastructure capable of delivering screening or an immunization programme. This includes trained personnel, equipment and laboratory facilities, information systems which determine who is eligible for the procedure and record uptake rates, and, in the case of immunization, a vaccine which is effective and safe. It can be seen then that the medical approach to health promotion can be a complex process, and may depend on the establishment of national programmes or guidelines.

Having screening or immunization facilities available is effective only if people can be persuaded to use them.

Evaluation

Evaluation of preventive procedures is based ultimately on a reduction in disease rates and associated mortality. This is a long-term process and a more popular measure capable of short-term evaluation is the increase in the percentage of the target population being screened or immunized.

In 1990 increased remuneration was introduced for GPs according to the achievement of targets for cervical cytology and

What methods can you think of that are used to increase the uptake of preventive services?

National campaigns may be launched but the one-to-one advice given to patients by health care workers is generally accepted as being more effective. Increasing uptake may thus depend on training health workers, having an efficient call system and offering screening at a convenient community location, such as in a mobile van.

immunization. This may have influenced the health promotion activities of some practices but it may have negative aspects. A King's Fund report on primary health care expresses some concern relating to: "the possible undermining of GPs' incentives to transmit to and gain from maximum amounts of information from their patients during opportunistic contacts, and the fact that the most disadvantaged communities may be comprised of individuals who are least able and/or willing to attend special health promotion clinics" (Taylor, 1991, p. 31).

 The medical approach is not always successful. Consider the example of cervical screening. The death rate from cervical cancer remains at a constant annual level of approximately 2000 per year despite a long established screening programme. What could account for the failure of this programme to reduce mortality?

You probably included some of the following:

■ Inadequate training of laboratory staff in detecting cancerous cell changes
■ Faults in the recall system
■ A more virulent virus
■ Inability to reach women most at risk
■ Low take up.

Behaviour change

Aims

This approach aims to encourage individuals to adopt healthy behaviours, which is seen as the key to improved health. Chapter 10 shows how making health-related decisions is a complex process and, unless a person is ready to take action, it is unlikely to be effective. As we saw in the previous chapter, seeking to influence or change health behaviour has long been part of health education.

The approach is popular because it views health as a property of individuals. It is then possible to assume that people can make real improvements to their health by choosing to change their lifestyle. Many of the targets in the national health strategy *The Health of the Nation* relate to changing behaviour. It is thus possible for Governments to demonstrate a commitment to health promotion without taking other action.

 Consider the reasons why people may not be able to put their knowledge of what constitutes a healthy diet into practice. Reasons include:

■ Lack of money
■ Family preferences
■ Lack of availability
■ Lack of cooking facilities.

It is clear that there is a complex relationship between individual behaviour, and social and environmental factors. Behaviour-change approaches have much in common with the free-market philosophy. Yet people come to the marketplace with very different abilities to purchase things, or to make lifestyle choices.

Methods

The behaviour-change approach is the bedrock of activity undertaken by the Health Education Authority (HEA). For example, the 'Look After Your Heart' campaign persuades people to desist from smoking, and adopt a healthy diet and regular exercise. This approach is targeted towards individuals, although mass means of communication may be used to reach them. It is most commonly an expert-led, top-down approach, which reinforces the divide between the expert who knows how to improve health and the general public who need education and advice. However, this is not inevitable. Interventions may be directed according to a client's stated needs when these have been identified.

Many health care workers educate their clients about health through the provision of information and one-to-one counselling. Patient education about a condition or medication may seek to ensure compliance, in other words, a behaviour change, or it may be more client directed and employ an educational approach.

Evaluation

Evaluating a health promotion intervention designed to change behaviour would appear to be a simple exercise. Has the health behaviour changed after the intervention? But there are two main problems: change may only become apparent over a long period, and it may be difficult to isolate any change as attributable to a health promotion intervention.

☞ The Stanford Three Community Study began in the USA in 1972. It sought to evaluate a year-long heart disease prevention project in two trial communities in California. One community received an intensive mass-media campaign; the second community received, in addition, screening and face to face health education; the third community was a control study which received no intervention. Both trial communities showed an increased knowledge of the risk factors associated with heart disease. Behavioural changes such as reduction in smoking and in dietary cholesterol were greater in the community receiving screening and health education. This study and a similar project in North Karelia in Finland, have shown that it is possible to bring about behaviour change. But it is difficult to prove unequivocally that observed changes were due to the health education project and not other factors, or the effect of being part of a research project.

Source: Tones et al., 1990.

The educational approach

Aims

The purpose of this approach is to provide knowledge and information, and to develop the necessary skills so that a person can make an informed choice about their health behaviour. The educational approach should be distinguished from a behaviour change approach in that it does not set out to persuade or motivate change in a particular direction. However, education *is* intended to have an outcome. This will be the client's voluntary choice and it may not be the one the health promoter would prefer.

The educational approach is based on a set of assumptions about the relationship between knowledge and behaviour: that by increasing knowledge, there will be a change in attitudes which may lead to changed behaviour. This ignores, however, not only the very real constraints that social and economic factors place on voluntary behaviour change, but also the complexities of health-related decision making (see Chapter 10).

Methods

Psychological theories of learning state that learning involves three aspects:

- Cognitive (information and understanding)
- Affective (attitudes and feelings)
- Behavioural (skills).

An educational approach to health promotion will provide information to help clients to make an informed choice about their health behaviour. It may also provide opportunities for clients to share and explore their attitudes to their own health. This may be through group discussion or one-to-one counselling. Educational programmes may also develop clients' decision-making skills through role plays or activities designed to explore options. Clients may take on roles or practise responses in "real-life" situations. For example, clients taking part in an alcohol programme may role-play situations where they are offered a drink. Educational programmes are usually led by a teacher or facilitator, although the issues for discussion may be decided by the clients.

Evaluation

Increases in knowledge are relatively easy to measure. Health education through mass media campaigns, one-to-one education and classroom-based work have all shown success in increasing information about health issues, or the awareness of risk factors for a disease. Information alone is, however, insufficient to change behaviour and, as we shall see in Chapter 10, even the desire and ability to change behaviour is no guarantee that the individual will do so.

Empowerment

Aims

This approach helps people to identify their own concerns and gain the skills and confidence to act upon them. It is unique in being based on a "bottom-up" strategy and calls for different skills from the health promoter. Instead of the expert role adopted by the other approaches, the health promoter becomes a facilitator. Their role is to act as a catalyst, getting things going, and then to withdraw from the situation.

When we talk of empowerment, we need to distinguish between *self*-empowerment and *community* empowerment. Self-empowerment is used in some cases to describe those approaches to promoting health which are based on counselling and which use non-directive client-centred approaches aimed at increasing people's control over their own lives.

Empowerment is also used to describe a way of working which increases people's power to change their "social reality". Chapter 9 includes a discussion of community development as a way of working which seeks to create active participating communities who are *empowered*, and able to challenge and change the world about them. This may or may not include political consciousness raising such as that advocated by the radical educationist, Paulo Freire (1972).

Methods

The emphasis on empowerment is probably familiar to many nurses developing a care plan with a patient, and to teachers working to raise pupils' self-esteem and to many other health promoters. They may call this approach client-centred or use terms such as advocacy or self-care. The role of the health promoter is to help clients to identify their health concerns and areas for change.

 A health visitor, in the course of carrying out visits to a new mother, finds the woman is bored and frustrated. The client identifies employment as the key to building her self-esteem. The health visitor works with the client, encouraging her confidence and finds the child a place in a day nursery.

Community development is a similar way of working to empower groups of people by identifying their concerns and working with them to plan a programme of action to address these concerns. Some health promoters have a specific remit to undertake community development work; most do not. Community development work is time-consuming and most health promoters have clearly defined priorities which take up all their time. Funding for this kind of work is invariably insecure and short term. The communication, planning and organizational skills necessary for this approach may not be included in professional training. For many health promoters, relinquishing the expert role may be difficult and uncomfortable. Ways of working with communities are discussed more fully in Chapter 9.

 Examples of health promotion through community development are:

1. Community development workers working with tenants on a housing estate to improve play space
2. Health promotion specialists using a variety of methods to identify health needs of residents in a particular area
3. Setting up groups to meet specific needs, e.g. a girls' group at a youth centre
4. Multi-lingual linkworkers running health sessions for Asian women.

Evaluation

Evaluation of such activity is problematic, partly because the process of empowerment and networking is typically long term. This makes it difficult to be certain that any changes detected are due to the intervention and not some other factor. In addition, positive results of such an approach may appear to be vague and hard to specify, especially when compared to outcomes used by other approaches, such as targets or changes in behaviour which are capable of being quantified. Evaluation includes the extent to which specific aims have been met (outcome evaluation) and the degree to which the group has gelled, or been empowered as a result of the intervention (process evaluation).

Social change

Aims

This approach which is sometimes referred to as radical health promotion, acknowledges the importance of the socio-economic environment in determining health. Its focus is at the policy or environmental level, and the aim is to bring about changes in the physical, social and economic environment which will have the effect of promoting health. This may be summed up in the phrase "to make the healthy choice the easier choice". A healthy choice is available, but to make it a realistic option for most people requires changes in its cost, availability or accessibility.

> **?** Several studies have shown that a healthy diet which includes fruit, vegetables, high-fibre foods and less fat and sugar, may cost up to a third more than the typical diet of a low income family (Cole-Hamilton and Lang, 1986). **What should be the focus of health promotion interventions on healthy eating?**
>
> You may have included some of the following:
>
> ■ Changes in pricing structures such as reducing the price of wholemeal bread compared to white bread
> ■ Working with food manufacturers and distributors to promote food labelling, making it easier for customers to identify low-fat, low-sugar foods
> ■ Farming subsidies which encourage the production of lean meat
> ■ The provision of healthy food in workplaces and hospitals
> ■ The re-introduction of nutritional standards for school meals which promote healthy food.

Methods

The social change or radical approach is targeted towards groups and populations, and involves a top-down method of working. Although there may be widespread consultation, the changes being sought are generally within organizations, and require commitment from the highest levels. We have already seen in the previous chapter how public health legislation has had an enormous impact on the nation's health. For such a policy to be successfully implemented, however, it has to be supported by a public who have been made aware of its importance.

For most health promotion workers, the scope for this type of activity will be more limited than for the traditional medical or behaviour change approaches. The necessary skills for working in this way, such as lobbying, policy planning, negotiating and implementation, may not be included in professional training. Working in such a way may be interpreted as beyond the brief of the job, too political or someone else's remit.

Are there parts of your work which are aimed at social change? Have you sought to influence policies and practices which affect health?

Organizational development, environmental health measures, economic or legislative activities and public policies on housing, education or the future of the NHS may all be examples of health promotion aimed at social change.

> **?** Table 5.1 uses the example of healthy eating to show how different approaches to health promotion will have different aims and use different methods.
>
> The "Health of the Nation" strategy identifies the following as key areas for health promotion: accidents, sexual health and AIDS, coronary heart disease and stroke, mental illness, and cancers. Consider how health promotion interventions in these areas will be affected by working with one of the five identified approaches to health promotion: medical, behaviour change, educational, empowerment, social change.
>
> ■ In each case what would working within this approach entail in terms of:
>   ■ Aims or focus?
>   ■ Methods?
>   ■ Worker/client relationship?
> ■ How would you evaluate your success using each approach?
> ■ With which approach would you feel most comfortable?

Table 5.1 Approaches to health promotion: the example of healthy eating.

Approach	Aims	Methods	Worker/client relationship
Medical	To identify those at risk from disease	Primary health care consultation, e.g. measurement of body mass index	Expert led. Passive, conforming client
Behaviour change	To encourage individuals to take responsibility for their own health and choose healthier lifestyles	Persuasion through one-to-one advice, Information, mass campaigns, e.g. 'Look After Your Heart' dietary messages	Expert led. Dependent client. Victim blaming ideology
Educational	To increase knowledge and skills about healthy lifestyles	Information Exploration of attitudes through small group work Development of skills, e.g. women's health group	May be expert led May also involve client in negotiation of issues for discussion
Empowerment	To work with clients or communities to meet their perceived needs	Advocacy Negotiation Networking Facilitation e.g. food co-op, fat women's group	Health promoter is facilitator. Client becomes empowered
Social change	To address inequalities in health based on class, race, gender, geography	Development of organizational policy, e.g. hospital catering policy Public health legislation, e.g. food labelling Lobbying Fiscal controls, e.g. subsidy to farmers to produce lean meat	Entails social regulation and is top-down

Models of health promotion

The above schema of different approaches to health promotion is primarily descriptive. It is what health promoters do, and it is possible to move in and out of different approaches depending on the situation. A more analytic means of identifying types of health promotion is to develop models of practice. A model is an abstract representation of reality, a conceptual framework. Models are generated by identifying criteria which govern practice such as "aims" or "degree of control". From this, it is possible to identify possibilities for practice.

Using a model can be helpful because it encourages you to think theoretically, and come up with new strategies and ways of working. It can also help you to prioritize and locate more or less desirable types of interventions.

There has been a proliferation of models in health promotion literature, with large areas of overlap but little consensus on terminology or underlying criteria. Thus we find that Beattie (1991) uses criteria of "mode of intervention" (authoritative–negotiated) and "focus of intervention" (individual–collective) to generate four models (see Figure 5.2 on page 95). Caplan and Holland (1990) use "theories of knowledge" and "theories of society" (see Figure 5.1 on page 94). The terminology for models also varies. Ewles and Simnett (1992) describe a "social change" approach to health promotion. French (1990) calls this "politics of health" (see Figure 5.3 on page 97), whilst Caplan and Holland (1990) distinguish between a radical model and a marxist model.

This can be extremely confusing for the reader. However, as Rawson (1992) points out, the debate about models of health promotion may be viewed as a healthy sign of an emerging occupation's concern to develop a sound theoretical basis for action.

1. Caplan and Holland (1990)

This model suggests there are essentially four paradigms or ways of looking at health promotion. These paradigms can be generated from two dimensions (see Figure 5.1 on page 94). The first dimension is concerned with the nature of knowledge. Knowledge is seen as based along a continuum which ranges from subjective approaches to understanding through to objective approaches. The second dimension relates to assumptions concerning the nature of society. These range from theories of radical change to theories of social regulation. When these two dimensions are put together it suggests four paradigms or perspectives of health promotion as illustrated in Figure 5.1.

Each quadrant represents a major approach to the understanding of health and the practice of health promotion. They are not necessarily exclusive but there will be situations when, to hold one position or approach, must preclude the adoption of other approaches. Each quadrant incorporates different theoretical and philosophical assumptions about society, concepts of health and the principal sources of health problems.

a. **The traditional perspective** relates to the medical and behaviour-change approaches described earlier. Knowledge lies with the experts and the emphasis is on information giving to bring about behaviour change.

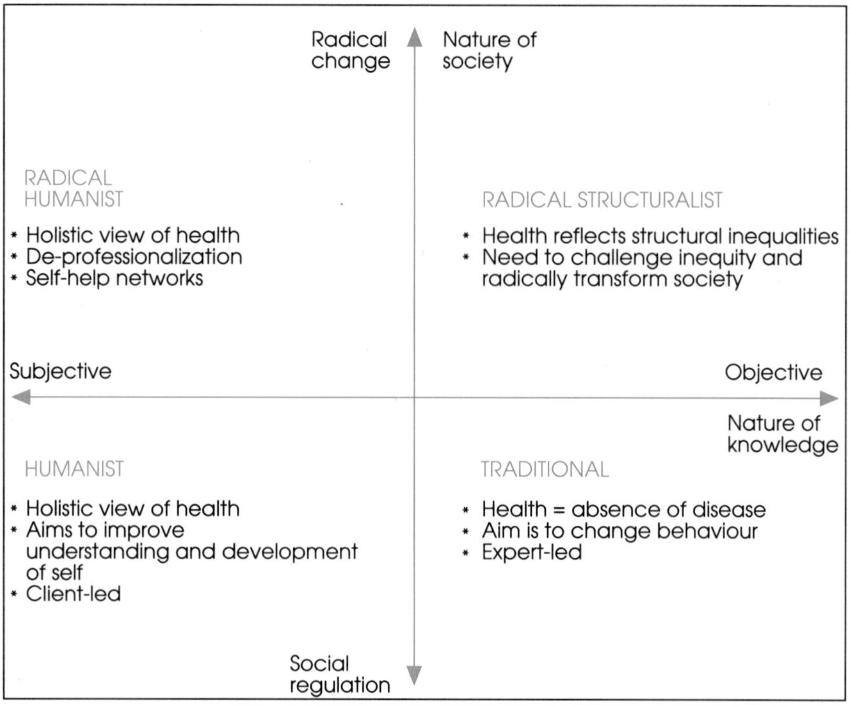

Figure 5.1 Four paradigms or perspectives of health promotion (adapted from Caplan and Holland, 1990).

b. **The humanist perspective** relates to the educational approach. Individuals are enabled to use their personal resources and skills to maximize their chances of developing what they consider to be a healthy lifestyle.

c. **The radical humanist perspective** relates to the empowerment approach. Health promotion is concerned to raise consciousness and part of the emphasis is on the exploration of personal responses to health issues. Alongside this, individuals are encouraged to form social, organizational and economic networks.

d. **The radical structuralist perspective** holds that structural inequalities are the cause of many health problems, and the role of health promotion is to address the relationship between health and social class.

2. Beattie (1991)

Beattie offers a structural analysis of the health promotion repertoire of approaches. He suggests there are four paradigms for health promotion (see Figure 5.2). These are generated from the dimensions of mode of intervention which ranges from authoritative (top-down and expert-led) to negotiated (bottom-up and valuing individual autonomy). The other dimension relates to focus of intervention which ranges from focus on the individual to a focus on the collective or group.

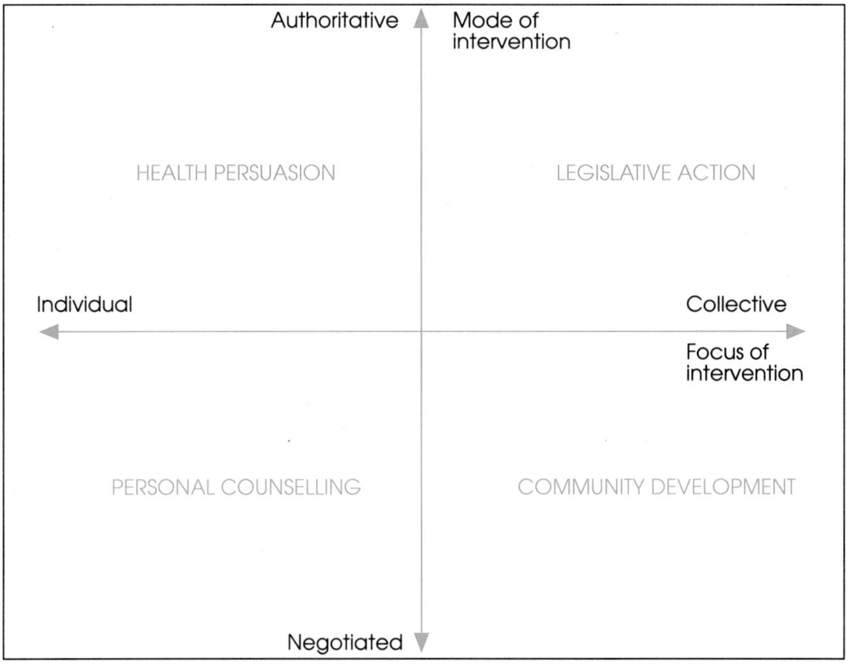

Figure 5.2 Strategies of health promotion (from Beattie, 1991).

Beattie's typology generates four strategies for health promotion. These are described in more detail in Chapter 7 on "The politics of health promotion" but briefly these are as follows.

a. **Health persuasion.** These are interventions directed at individuals and led by professionals. An example is a primary health care worker encouraging a pregnant woman to stop smoking.

b. **Legislative action**. These are interventions led by professionals but intended to protect communities. An example is lobbying for a ban on tobacco advertising.

c. **Personal counselling.** These interventions are client led and focus on personal development. The health promoter is a facilitator rather than expert. An example is a youth worker working with young people who helps them to identify their health needs and then works with them one-to-one or through group work to increase their confidence and skills.

d. **Community development**. These interventions, in a similar way to personal counselling, seek to empower or enhance the skills of a group or local community.

Each of these strategies corresponds to a different political perspective as illustrated below. Thus conservative and reformist perspectives see health promotion as attempting to correct or repair what is seen as a deficit in the conservative perspective, or an aspect of deprivation in the reformist perspective. These perspectives give rise to authoritative and prescriptive approaches.

Libertarian and radical perspectives see health promotion as seeking to empower or enfranchise individuals as in the libertarian perspective. The radical perspective, in addition, seeks to mobilize and emancipate communities.

Beattie's model is a useful one for health promoters because it identifies a clear framework for deciding a strategy, and yet reminds them that the choice of these interventions is influenced by social and political perspectives.

3. French and Adams (1986)

French and Adams propose a triphasic hierarchy of models. Phase 1 is a behaviour change model which includes medical, behaviour change and educational approaches. Phase 2 is the self-empowerment model which aims to increase individual autonomy. Phase 3 is the collective action model.

French and Adams reject typologies which use dimensions arguing that health promotion encompasses too many philosophical and methodological issues affecting the nature and practice of health promotion to be plotted in this way. Their model is therefore a map which considers aims, models of health, models of humanity, models of society, models of education, examples of methods, and examples of evaluation criteria. Some of the implications for practice can be illustrated (see Figure 5.3).

> **?** **Consider what models of humanity, society and education might be suggested by each of the following models:**
>
> ■ Behaviour change
> ■ Self-empowerment
> ■ Collective action.

French and Adams argue that many health promoters practise first, and then attempt to explain and justify their interventions, whereas a theory for health promotion should come first. Health promoters need to be clear about the values and assumptions which underpin different approaches to health promotion. French and Adams state that collective action is the most desirable form of health promotion because it locates health as a social issue. In this sense, their model differs from those of other authors by stating a preferred position, and suggesting that health promotion is not merely a technical and eclectic area of study.

In 1990 French developed a further typology which he argues is a more "sophisticated and understandable scheme" which can be used by pragmatic health promoters. In this typology he identifies four models: disease management; disease prevention; health

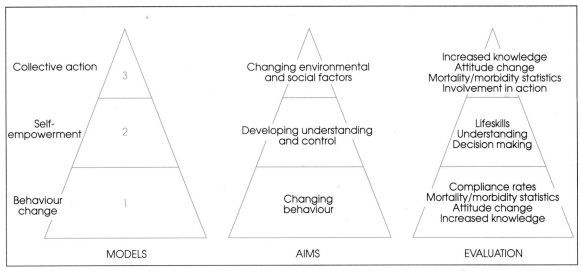

Figure 5.3 A tri-phasic map of health education (adapted from French and Adams, 1986).

education; and politics of health, which reflect the multi-faceted nature of health promotion (see Figure 5.4).

4. Tannahill (Downie et al., 1990)

This model of health promotion is widely accepted by health care workers. Tannahill talks of three overlapping spheres of activity: health education; health protection; and prevention. Tannahill's diagrammatic representation (Figure 5.5) shows how different approaches relate to each other in an all-inclusive process termed health promotion.

The model is primarily descriptive of what goes on in practice. It is useful for the health promoter to see the potential in other areas

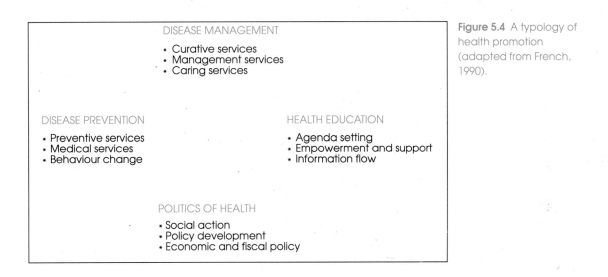

Figure 5.4 A typology of health promotion (adapted from French, 1990).

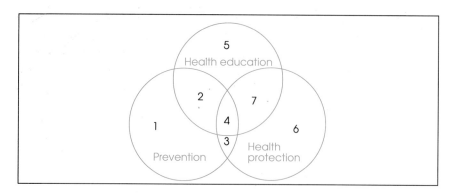

Figure 5.5 Tannahill's model of health promotion (from Downie *et al.*, 1990).
1. Preventive services, e.g. immunization, cervical screening, hypertension case finding, developmental surveillance, use of nicotine chewing gum to aid smoking cessation.
2. Preventive health education, e.g. smoking cessation advice and information.
3. Preventive health protection, e.g. fluoridation of water.
4. Health education for preventive health protection, e.g. lobbying for seat-belt legislation.
5. Positive health education, e.g. lifeskills work with young people.
6. Positive health protection, e.g. workplace smoking policy.
7. Health education aimed at positive health protection, e.g. lobbying for a ban on tobacco advertising.

of activity, but the areas of distinction and overlap can cause disagreement.

5. Tones (Tones et al., 1990)

Tones makes a simple equation that health promotion is an overall process of healthy public policy × health education (see Figure 5.6). In his model health education consists of two strands of education

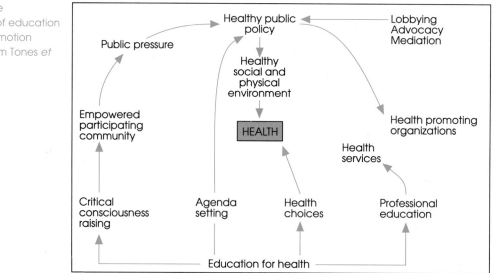

Figure 5.6 The contribution of education to health promotion (adapted from Tones *et al.*, 1990).

and information to enable individuals to make choices. Alongside this, health education also sets an agenda and raises consciousness to create pressure for a healthy public policy. The model assumes that both strands are necessary. Changes in the social environment achieved through a healthy public policy will produce changes in individuals. The support of individuals is also necessary for implementing environmental change. Empowerment, as opposed to prevention or a radical–political approach is the main aim of health promotion in Tones' model. Working for empowerment enhances individual autonomy and enables individuals, groups and communities to take more control over their lives.

Conclusion

A number of quite different activities are subsumed under the label "health promotion". Attempts to organize these activities into different categories has generated a plethora of models and typologies. The most obvious starting point is to describe the variety of current practice and this is the approach taken at the beginning of this chapter. However, there are limitations to this method and it may be criticized as being insufficiently analytical. Theorists who have taken this one step further have identified key criteria which serve to locate different forms of practice, both existing and potential. Adopting a more analytical approach enables judgements to be made about more and less desirable forms of practice, and opens up these judgements for debate. If health promotion is to progress as a discipline and an activity in its own right, a strong theoretical framework is necessary.

The search to clarify models and typologies of practice may appear to be academic and unrelated to the "here and now" of your activities to promote health. However, we would argue that for practice to grow beyond a reactive response to demands made by others, practitioners need to have an idea of all available options. It is only when we can contemplate different ways of promoting health that we can make judgements as to what is possible and what is preferable. Recognizing that the two are not always synonymous may be frustrating in the short term, but must in the long term contribute towards the effectiveness and efficiency of health promotion.

Questions for further discussion

- Which approach(es) to health promotion do you adopt in your work?
- What are the most important reasons for adopting your approach(es)?

■ Which typology or model of health promotion do you find most helpful in providing a theoretical framework with which to analyse your health promotion activities?

Summary

This chapter has examined five different approaches to health promotion: the medical or preventive approach; the behaviour change or lifestyles approach; the educational approach; the empowerment and community development approach; the social change or radical approach. In practice, the edges between them may be blurred. However, they do differ in significant ways. They encompass different assumptions concerning the nature of health, society and change. The preferred methods of intervention, necessary skills and means of evaluation all differ. Many health promoters will find that the approach they adopt is dictated, in part at least, by their job role and functions. This chapter stresses the importance of examining your approach to health promotion and identifying any changes you may wish to make.

Further reading

Ewles L and Simnett I (1992) *Promoting Health*, Chichester, Wiley.

Chapter 3 provides a short and straightforward guide to approaches to health promotion and identifies their aims and values.

Rawson D (1992) "The growth of health promotion theory and its radical reconstruction", in Bunton R and Macdonald G (1992) *Health Promotion: Disciplines and Diversity*, London, Routledge.

A powerful argument for the importance of theory in developing health promotion practice. This chapter examines the multidisciplinary roots to health promotion theory and practice.

Tones K, Tilford S and Robinson Y (1990) *Health Education: Effectiveness and Efficiency,* London, Chapman & Hall.

Chapter 1 explores the values underpinning three different models of health promotion: radical–political model; self-empowerment; and preventive model.

References

Beattie A (1991) "Knowledge and control in health promotion: a test case for social policy and social theory", in Gabe J, Calnan M and Bury M *The Sociology of the Health Service*, London, Routledge.

Caplan R and Holland R (1990) "Rethinking health education theory" *Health Education Journal*, **49**, 10–12.

Cole-Hamilton I and Lang T (1986) *Tightening Belts: A Report on the Impact of Poverty on Food*, London, Food Commission.

Downie RS, Fyfe C and Tannahill A (1990) Health Promotion: Models and Values, Oxford, Oxford Medical Publications.

Ewles L and Simnett I (1992) *Promoting Health*, London, Scutari Press.

French J (1990) "Models of health education and promotion", *Health Education Journal*, **49**, 1.

French J and Adams L (1986) "From analysis to synthesis", *Health Education Journal*, **45**, 2.

Rawson D (1992) "The growth of health promotion theory and its rational reconstruction" in Bunton R and Macdonald G (eds) *Health Promotion: Disciplines and Diversity*, London, Routledge.

Taylor D (1991) *Developing Primary Care: Opportunities for the 1990s*, London, King's Fund.

Tones K, Tilford S and Robinson Y (1990) *Health education; Effectiveness and Efficiency*, London, Chapman & Hall.

SECTION 2
Dilemmas in Practice

This section addresses some of the practice issues for health promoters, in particular the ethical and political dilemmas which face a reflective practitioner. Two strategies which are investigated are community development and behaviour change. How can health promoters work with communities and what are the strengths and limitations of a community development approach? What influences health behaviour and how can we help people to change?

E*thical issues in health promotion*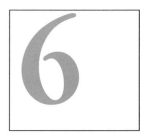

Overview

Health promotion involves working to improve people's health. This requires a series of value judgements: about what better health means for the individual and society; and about whether, when and how to make a health promotion intervention. This book has used the perspectives of social science to help you to explore your role and aims in health promotion. In this chapter we consider some of the prevailing problems for a health promoter from a philosophical perspective. In particular the chapter focuses on the limits to individual freedoms and how these are balanced against the health of the community. The chapter outlines the key ethical principles of beneficence ("doing good"), justice, and respect for persons and their autonomy.

Key points
- The importance of ethical decision making in health promotion
- Duties in health promotion
- The individual and the common good
- Definitions of autonomy and its limits
- Justice in health promotion
- Professional codes of practice

The need for a philosophy of health promotion

Debate in health promotion has centred on discussion of practice and some attempts to develop a theoretical base. However, according to Seedhouse (1988), there has been little discussion concerning the philosophy of health and yet it is an essential part of the way in which we understand the world.

Health promotion involves decisions and choices that affect other people which require judgements to be made about whether particular courses of action are right or wrong. There are no definite ways to behave. Health promotion is, according to Seedhouse (1988), "a moral endeavour". Philosophical debate helps to clarify what it is that one believes in most and how one wants to run one's life. It can and does help practitioners to reflect on the principles of practice, and thus to make practical judgements about whether to intervene and which strategies to adopt.

Philosophy has three main branches:

- Logic – the development of reasoned argument
- Epistemology – the debate and discussion of truths such as the meaning of health
- Ethics – the formal study of the principles on which moral rules and values are based.

Morals refer to those beliefs about how people "ought" to behave. These debates about right and wrong, good and bad, and duty are part of everyday discourse. Is it wrong to tell a lie? Is it justified to kill another? Is it our duty to look after ageing parents? Judgements about the morality of these actions may derive from our personal values and moral beliefs which derive from: religion, culture, ideology, or professional codes of practice or social etiquette; the law; or our life experience. The function of ethical theory is not to provide answers but to inform these judgements and help people work out whether certain courses of action are right or wrong, and whether one ought to take a certain action.

Most ethical theories fall into two types – deontological and consequential. Deontology comes from the Greek word *deontos* meaning duty. Deontologists hold that we have a *duty* to act in accordance with certain universal moral rules. Consequential ethics are based on the premise that whether an action is right or wrong depends on its end result.

Duty

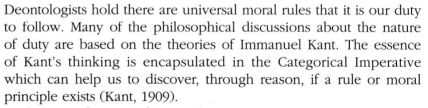

This example centres on the duty to respect life and highlights some of the difficulties that can arise from carrying out this duty.

There is in medical care a commonly accepted doctrine of "acts and omissions" which states that if a person fails to perform an action that would prevent negative consequences s/he is morally less blameworthy than if s/he performed an action that resulted in the same consequences.

Deontologists hold there are universal moral rules that it is our duty to follow. Many of the philosophical discussions about the nature of duty are based on the theories of Immanuel Kant. The essence of Kant's thinking is encapsulated in the Categorical Imperative which can help us to discover, through reason, if a rule or moral principle exists (Kant, 1909).

The major features of Kant's theory are:

1. Act as if your action in each circumstance is to become law for everyone, yourself included, in the future. In other words, if everyone always behaved this way, would the overall effect be good? If it would, then this is the rule to apply in all similar situations. The biblical "Do unto others as you would they do unto you" becomes a universal moral imperative.
2. Always treat human beings as "ends in themselves" and never merely as "means". A moral rule then is one that respects all people.

Deontological theories make decision making apparently easy because, as long as we obey the rules, then we must be doing the right thing, regardless of the consequences.

Many health care workers have codes of practice which require the fulfilment of duties. For example, the 1992 code of practice from the UK Central Council of Nursing, Midwifery and Health Visiting states the duty to respect life, the duty to care, and the duty to do no harm. Kant would have added "the duty to be truthful in all declarations is a sacred, unconditional command of reason, and not to be limited by any expediency" (Kant, 1909). Yet health care workers can probably think of numerous situations where a duty to tell the truth comes into conflict with other ethical principles such as avoiding harm.

Ethical principles are becoming as important for health promoters as they are for doctors and nursing staff.

? **The Society for Health Education and Promotion Specialists (SHE/PS) (1990) includes these principles among others in its code of conduct. That practitioners have a duty to:**

- ■ "not participate in health education/promotion activities for which the practitioner is not adequately trained or competent"
- ■ "not be involved in providing services designed solely to meet the demands of income generation or other subsidiary goals at the expense of meeting demonstrable health needs".

How would you respond in each of these situations?
- ■ A member of staff refuses to undertake aspects of their job description for which they are not properly trained and therefore not "competent".
- ■ To generate much-needed income the health promotion department's mobile health unit decides to charge the public for cholesterol testing. The health authority does not regard cholesterol testing as beneficial and fears that GPs will be overburdened by patients made unnecessarily anxious by the cholesterol testing.

There is an increasing trend towards sponsorship for health promotion activities. This ranges from the sponsorship of apparently healthy activities such as the Olympic Games by Coca Cola to health research sponsored by a tobacco company trust to the sponsorship of health information by drug companies, sanitary wear manufacturers or a local health food shop. Is sponsorship compatible with health promotion? The code of practice of the Society of Health Education/Promotion Specialists suggests that sponsorship is acceptable when it comes from enterprises compatible with health promotion principles and practices, and when the acceptance of income does not divert the practitioners from meeting more demonstrable health needs.

(cont.)
In 1992 Dr Nigel Cox was convicted of murdering his patient Lilian Boyes who was suffering a lingering and painful death. Dr Cox administered a lethal dose of potassium chloride. This was regarded as active killing, although the General Medical Council decided not to strike Dr Cox off the medical register.

In 1992 medical staff stopped feeding Tony Bland, a young man crushed into a permanent vegetative state by the Hillsborough football disaster. This action was regarded as withholding life saving treatment and morally acceptable.

Both acts had brought about the same consequence – the death of a patient. Is there a moral distinction, in your view, between killing and letting die? Must human life be preserved regardless of its quality?

> **?** **Which of the following would you find acceptable?**
>
> - A curriculum pack for schools on puberty sponsored by a sanitary wear manufacturer
> - A leaflet on safer sex sponsored by the London Rubber Company, manufacturers of condoms
> - A research project on healthy lifestyles supported by a tobacco company trust
> - An education project for convicted drink-drivers sponsored by a brewery group
> - An information handbook on local support services which includes advertisements from local businesses.

Consequentialism and utilitarianism

The other classical school of ethics is known as consequentialism, of which utilitarianism is its best known branch. Consequentialism differs from deontological theories because it is concerned with ends and not only means. The utilitarian principle is that a person should always act in such a way that will produce more good or benefits than disadvantages. Utilitarians such as John Stuart Mill and Jeremy Bentham aimed for the greatest good or pleasure for the greatest number of people. Utilitarians can thus respond to all moral dilemmas by reviewing the facts and weighing up the consequences of alternative courses of action. This can, of course, prove difficult. What exactly is a good end? How does one predict whether an outcome will be favourable? One of the main problems with utilitarianism is that, if the aim of all actions is to achieve the greatest good, does this justify harm or injustice to a few if society benefits? Smoking restrictions offer an example where the health of society takes precedence over the right of the individual to smoke.

This raises key philosophical and political questions about freedom and its limits. Should the interests of the majority always take precedence over those of the individual? In Chapter 4 we saw that some writers have expressed concern over "social engineering" in health promotion and that Government intervention has risked becoming Government intrusion. Many interventions are not requested or desired, yet may be enforced by law.

> **Consider these examples of a possible healthy public policy and whether, in your view, they are ethical.**
>
> - Compulsory use of seat belts for front and back seat drivers and passengers
> - Fluoridation of tap water
> - Subsidy of lead-free petrol
> - Smoke-free zones on public transport
> - Complete ban on drinking and driving
> - Compulsory testing of all visitors to UK for HIV infection.

Ethical principles

Ethical principles can help to clarify the decisions that have to be taken at work. Sometimes decisions may be guided by trying to do the best for the most number of people, at other times they may be guided by an overriding concern for peoples' right to determine their own lives; and sometimes decisions may be guided by other ethical principles or a professional code of conduct.

There are four widely accepted ethical principles (Beauchamp and Childress, 1989):

Respect for autonomy (a respect for the rights of individuals and their right to determine their lives)
Beneficence (doing good)
Non-maleficence (doing no harm)
Justice (being fair and equitable).

These principles provide a framework for consistent moral decision making. However, situations rarely involve a single option, but can encapsulate increasingly complex and sometimes conflicting choices between these principles. Seedhouse (1988) has developed these principles into an ethical grid which helps provide the health promoter with an easy-to-follow guide on which to ground their work on moral principles (see Figure 6.1).

Autonomy

Autonomy derives from the Greek word *autonomous* meaning self-rule. It refers to a person's capacity to choose freely for themselves and be able to direct their own life. Since people do not exist in isolation from each other, there will be restrictions on individual autonomy and the autonomous person has a sense of responsibility: they cannot do entirely as they like. Beyond this, traditional notions of liberal individualism see autonomy as essential to all human beings. It is only constrained by:

Reason and the ability to make rational choices
The ability to understand one's environment
The ability to act on one's environment.

In addition, a person needs to be free from pressures such as fear and want, and have the personal and social circumstances to make any chosen action possible.

Autonomy must, therefore, be thought of not as an absolute but as attainable, to a greater or lesser extent. Not everyone has autonomy. When a person's capacity for rationality is affected in some way, decisions are often taken on their behalf on the basis that "they do not know what's best for them". Thus people with

Figure 6.1 The Ethical Grid (from Seedhouse, 1988). The limit to the use of the grid is that it should be used honestly to seek to enable the enhancing potentials of people.

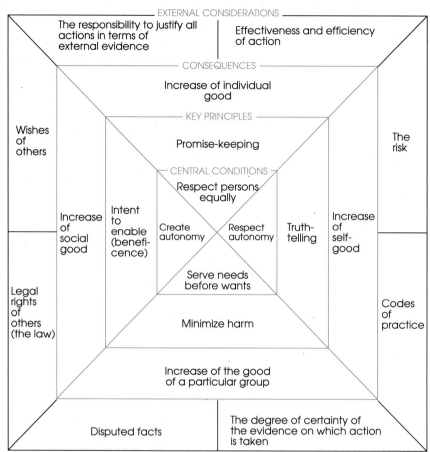

learning difficulties or mental illness, young children and older people with mental confusion are often assumed to be unable to make a rational choice.

There has been widespread debate in recent years over the rights of people with learning disabilities (or difficulties). For example, the decision of a court to allow the sterilization of a 17-year-old girl denied this young woman the right to have a child. However, this was considered in her best interests rather than the possible trauma of pregnancy and childbirth or abortion, for which it was considered she would not be prepared. It was also deemed in the best interests of a possible child who would not be able to be brought up by the young woman. In another case, a young woman was put on the Pill as it was deemed she would not be able to make rational decisions about contraception and could not be prevented from having sexual intercourse.

> "Because parents are uncertain or in conflict as to what retarded adolescents' adult roles will be, they are unsure how to prepare teenagers for transition to adulthood. They are more likely to encourage dependency, obedience and childlike behaviour, rather than independence, self-direction, assumption of responsibility and sexual awareness" (Craft, 1987).

In these situations, what do we mean by autonomy? In part we must mean respecting our clients as persons and helping them to cope with the consequences of their choices. Seedhouse (1988) makes a distinction between creating autonomy and respecting autonomy, which he regards as the central conditions when working for health.

Creating autonomy is making an effort to improve the quality of a person's autonomy by trying to enhance what that person is able to do. In health promotion work, this is often called empowerment. It may involve information to enable clients to make choices or developing the clients' skills in analysing situations and making decisions through increasing self-awareness and assertiveness. As we have stated elsewhere in this book, it is of prime importance in health promotion practice to recognize the limits to individual autonomy, and that social and economic circumstances can constrain individual health choices. Health promoters must avoid victim blaming and seeing people as solely responsible for their own ill health.

Respecting autonomy is agreeing to the wishes of the individual and respecting their chosen direction, whether or not it is approved. Creating and respecting autonomy are closely related. A person cannot express a free wish if they are not aware of the possibilities open to them and thus it may, in some circumstances, be ethically justifiable not to respond to a client's expressed wishes but to attempt to open up other options.

Respecting clients' autonomy can be difficult for health promoters. There is often a tendency to give advice, to offer information or to persuade a client to change their behaviour. The challenge is to accept a role of partner and enabler rather than expert and controller. Ewles and Simnett (1992) identify three common ways in which health promoters hinder rather than respect their clients' autonomy:

- By imposing their own solutions to the clients' problems
- By instructing clients on what to do because s/he takes too long to work it out for him or herself
- By dismissing the client's ideas without providing an adequate explanation or the opportunity to try them out

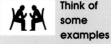 **Think of some examples** from your work when you have attempted to create autonomy in your clients so that they are able to express their wishes and wants.

At what point did you decide that the client is autonomous and to *respect* their wishes?

Chapter 9 explores a community development way of working which seeks to empower people with regard to their own health agenda. It explores this dilemma of control and autonomy, and to what extent community development workers impose, collaborate with, or genuinely facilitate local or community health needs.

Perhaps the starkest example of the ethical problems associated with respecting autonomy is that which confronts the health worker when a patient or client chooses not to follow advice or treatment which is known to be beneficial (see Figure 6.2). It would seem straightforward that this is the client's right and the health worker should respect the client's autonomy in choosing such a decision, if the client is properly informed and understands any risks involved. However, the health worker is committed to "doing good" and may feel it is their duty to persuade the client. This is particularly so if the client's decision has implications for other people. Certainly this is paternalistic and putting the health worker's need to do good above the client's wish for autonomy.

? A patient who has undergone heart bypass surgery continues to smoke after the operation.

■ Is it justifiable to refuse further treatment?
■ What factors do you take into account in making your judgement?

This extract suggests the following:

" . . . a doctor who takes seriously his self-imposed and professional obligation to benefit his patient ought to treat the patient if that is what the patient on reflection wants him to do, if some treatment is available which will provide net benefit to the patient . . . Of course that in no way prevents the doctor from advising that the most effective way of regaining and maintaining health is to alter one's lifestyle in the relevant way. But coercion will generally be contraindicated by the requirement to respect people's autonomy, and withdrawal of care from those who reject one's advice will generally be contraindicated by a doctor's personally and professionally undertaken duty of care, or obligation of beneficence" (Gillon, 1990, p. 34).

Respecting autonomy involves respecting another person's rights and dignity such that a person reaches a maximum level of fulfilment as a human being. In the context of health promotion and health care this means that the relationship with the patient or client is based on a respect for him or her as a person, and with individual rights. It follows we must then see them as 'whole people' – with physical, social, emotional and spiritual needs – as fundamentally equal and also as unique individuals.

Rights in relation to health care are usually taken to include:

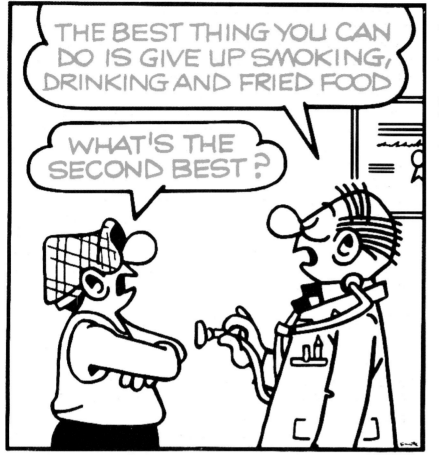

Figure 6.2 Andy Capp cartoon used in the Health Education Authority's *Look After Your Heart* campaign. Reproduced with kind permission of Mirror Group Newspapers. Distributed by North America Syndicate.

- The right to information
- The right to privacy and confidentiality
- The right to appropriate care and treatment.

Health workers are often placed in the position of deciding whether to inform patients or relatives of an adverse prognosis. Although the patients' right to information is usually considered paramount, there are occasions when the health workers' duty of beneficence – to do good and avoid harm – may outweigh this right. Placing individual rights as central does protect the dignity of the individual and their needs. However, if the maintenance of such rights threatens the protection of society, then the right is not inviolable, merely desirable.

> **Parents, pupils or staff of a school may wish to know of the presence of an HIV-positive child or member of staff, either out of concern about a possible health risk to themselves or their child, or because they believe a sharing of such information would enable them to provide better care and support for the child.**
>
> Should this information be disclosed?

This situation raises issues about the right to information and the right to privacy. Most authorities would emphasize respect for the individual's right to privacy. As there is no health risk attached to the presence of an HIV-positive person if good hygiene is routinely applied, there is no harm in keeping HIV status confidential. Indeed, the possible harm to the individual that might arise in the case of disclosure from possible discrimination or isolation outweighs these understandable concerns.

Beneficence and non maleficence

Frankena (1963) suggests that beneficence means doing or promoting good as well as preventing, removing and avoiding evil or harm.

> 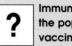 **Immunization is effective only if a high level of immunity is achieved in the population. Is it ethical for individuals to be persuaded to take up a vaccine if its safety is in doubt?**
>
> After considering a response to this dilemma, note the example of congenital rubella syndrome.
>
> Rubella vaccine is given to children of both sexes at about 15 months as part of the measles, mumps and rubella (MMR) combined immunization programme. Unless 90% of children are immunized, girls who are not vaccinated are likely to reach child-bearing age without a natural immunity. Before MMR, when the vaccine was given only to girls at puberty, this situation would have been unlikely.
>
> The intent to promote the health of the community may thus have adverse consequences for a small minority of women.

In such circumstances the duty to care has to be extended to include the concept of informed consent. The individual must be informed, and understand the information and implications of any action which is taken to be beneficial. In this way the health worker can be said to be avoiding harm.

In the field of drug education, harm minimization is increasingly adopted as a way of working. This is perhaps more realistic than the encompassing principle of doing no harm. The health care

---

What is the nature of 'goodness" in health promotion work?

For the health promoter doing good may be said to be improving the health and well-being of individuals or groups. Traditional preventive health education may be regarded as a protective beneficence which prevents harm in the long term. A dilemma arises for the practitioner when the outcome or consequence of an action which is deemed "good" for the health of the community may involve harm for the individual. Immunization, regarded as a key element in preventive health education, poses this sort of dilemma.

worker recognizes that the client may not wish to change their behaviour, and therefore seeks to encourage a safer way of life and reduce its harm. Drug workers may give clients clean needles, condoms, and provide information about emergency first aid to reduce the risks of HIV infection or accidents.

Justice

Philosophers suggest three versions of justice:

■ The fair distribution of scarce resources
■ Respect for individual and group rights
■ Following morally acceptable laws.

Thus justice requires that people are treated equally. But what is meant by equal? Does it mean according to equal need? Or according to equal ability? Or according to equal contribution?

For example, the equal distribution of resources can mean different things. It could mean that resources should be distributed equally in mathematical terms. Or should they be distributed according to how much was contributed – thus those that have and can put in most get out most? Or should we apply the Marxist adage "From each according to his ability, to each according to their need"? The NHS was established on the basis of free medical care to all those who need it. In an era of scarce resources, demand far exceeds supply. Need is an obvious criterion for distributing care but it is not sufficient. Tudor Hart whose inverse care law was described in Chapter 2 observed that those who needed health care most received least (Tudor Hart, 1971). As we shall see in Chapter 11, although we may use some objective measurement for the assessment of individual health needs, such as the ability to self-care or to perform certain tasks, this does not overcome the subjective value judgement that is involved in making these decisions. In recent years, health economists have tried to establish some other sort of objective and measurable criteria to compare competing claims – possibly the relative financial costs of treatment or an assessment made on QALYs, which are described in Chapter 3.

Issues of justice are glaringly evident in health promotion. We read earlier the evidence of wide differences in health status between different groups in society. Whilst the health promoter may be unable to alter society's inequities they may, nevertheless, be able to work on programmes which acknowledge that people's potential for health is different and which avoid victim blaming.

Being fair to everyone might seem to suggest adopting public health measures which iron out differences in resources, health care or environmental quality. Yet any kind of state intervention means addressing the issue of individual rights versus the common good. For instance, would it be just that top wage earners should pay 50% income tax to finance public spending on health and welfare? The following chapter examines different political perspectives on health promotion, and the fundamental differences between right and left of the political spectrum towards health and welfare.

Screening

The example of screening illustrates the complexities of ethical decision making and how attempting to follow the key ethical principles of doing good and avoiding harm is not a simple process.

Most preventive services are offered with an explicit promise that they will do some good and an implicit understanding that they will do no harm. Yet what is the nature of that good? Screening, for example, only tells someone they are healthy at the present time. A negative result does not mean that illness will not develop the following year. Screening cannot promise a good outcome. Early detection can mean more effective or less radical treatment in some cases, but there may be no medical benefit and no treatment available. This is currently the case with HIV infection. Hopes that the drug AZT would arrest the progression of HIV infection have not been confirmed by research.

> **?** Consider these points in relation to a screening process with which you are familiar. Do you conclude that screening is of benefit, avoids harm and respects all persons equally?
>
> 1. Screening is never wholly routine and inclusive. It is targeted to identified risk groups and therefore excludes certain categories of people, usually on the grounds of age.
> 2. Screening is spaced due to economic considerations and therefore people may develop the disease in the intervening period.
> 3. The screening process may foster anxieties.
> 4. The screening process may be uncomfortable or painful.
> 5. The call and recall procedures may be poorly handled and the informing of results may take some time.
> 6. Screening uses high sensitivity methods which can result in a high number of false positive results. These people will be subjected to unnecessary worry and distress.
> 7. Screening uses methods which are less than 100% specific – therefore some people will go away falsely reassured.

Ethically, screening represents the tension between beneficence and non-maleficence. It is seen as a good but is not without harm. Duncan (1990) argues that screening highlights the importance of informed consent, and clients being aware of the benefits and disadvantages. Unfortunately the pressure to ensure adequate take-up and to demonstrate success of a service means screening is often "sold" to the public and they are not fully informed. Duncan concludes that health promoters must ask:

- Are we enabling our clients' participation in screening?
- Are we helping to put this episode and any resulting advice in the context of their lives?
- Are we selling what is on offer in such a way that it is quite clear what is being sold? (Duncan, 1990).

Information giving

The process of information giving in health promotion also involves complex ethical decisions. Seedhouse (1988) identifies truth telling and promise keeping as principles which the health promoter should hold onto when deliberating a course of action. As we saw earlier the patient's right to information and the health promoter's duty to tell the truth may conflict with the duty of beneficence.

"Do-gooding" may not in fact be sought or wanted by the client. As we saw in Chapter 4, the essential nature of health education is that it is based on a principle of voluntarism. It should neither seek to coerce or persuade, but to facilitate informed choice.

Many health promotion practitioners would state their intention to empower their clients and facilitate informed choices. It is, however, often easier when convinced of the "good" of an action to select the information or evidence in order to persuade. Campbell (1990) suggests that persuasion is acceptable only if a true picture of various aspects is presented. All education, he argues, involves some persuasion, and it is too simplistic to suggest that a desire to empower and create autonomy rules out persuasion. This means, however, that the health promoter must ensure the client *seeks* advice and help, and is not persuaded against their will. Secondly, the health education must be based on evidence, and be free from political control or vested interests.

> **Is it ethical to carry out opportunistic health education in primary health care?**
>
> Consider the example of a patient who goes to their GP with back pain. The doctor takes the opportunity for some health education, and takes the patient's blood pressure and family history. The patient had neither sought this nor was she made aware beforehand of the implications should raised blood pressure be found.
>
> The patient has not freely chosen to have her blood pressure checked in this way. Although she gave her consent, it might not be regarded as fully informed.

> **☞ Consider the example of healthy eating. The Health Education Authority "Look After Your Heart" campaign recommends the reduction of saturated fat in the diet. Yet the evidence is far from clear that those with normal cholesterol levels would reduce their risk of heart disease by reducing their fat consumption. According to Le Fanu (1987) the medical profession is guilty of misusing scientific evidence and selectively interpreting data. Although this debate is widely aired in medical journals, the public does not have access to the debate nor the experience to make a decision for themselves as a single message is promoted.**

Political pressure can make it difficult for the public to make an informed decision. Farming interests have meant that concerns about food safety have been slow to become public knowledge. For example, the Department of Health informed the food processing industry in 1988 of the dangers of salmonella in eggs after a major increase in notifications of salmonella poisoning since 1981. However, it took a statement by Edwina Currie, the Junior Health Minister that "most egg production in this country is sadly infected with salmonella" for the information to become known to the public. Edwina Currie subsequently lost her job.

> **?** Because the knowledge base of health promotion is changing, there are few areas where recommendations can be made on a factual basis. Kemm (1991) has described health promotion as lacking rigour and based on "best available opinion". It is possible to think of numerous examples in recent years where information on the risks or benefits of certain behaviours has changed.
>
> ■ The contraceptive pill is now contra-indicated for a wider group of women
> ■ The importance of reducing saturated fat for those with normal cholesterol levels is disputed
> ■ Potatoes are no longer thought to be fattening but a good bulk food and source of fibre
> ■ Moderate amounts of alcohol are now thought to have a beneficial effect on the heart.
>
> Should the public be made aware of debates over the evidence for health promotion advice? Should interventions be employed when the evidence for their effectiveness is in doubt?

Conclusion

Do practitioners whose work involves decisions affecting the lives of others engage in a moral deliberation about the best course of action? In general, most combine features of utility and deontology. They respect autonomy, try to be honest and fair, and avoid victim blaming. At the same time they try to achieve the best overall solution to any given situation. Yet situations can involve complex layers of decision making involving many ethical dilemmas. Screening, for example, a frequently unchallenged linchpin of preventive health education, raises key issues about its benefits for an individual versus the increase of the social good as well as questions about the extent to which screening is honestly presented. Before we can make any sort of ethical judgement we need to be clear about the values and principles which underpin our actions. If we return to the question asked earlier in this chapter, what do we mean by doing good and avoiding harm? Because ethical reflection involves deliberating on so many aspects, the Ethical Grid (Figure 6.1) developed by Seedhouse (1988) and commented on by Ewles and Simnett (1992) is extremely valuable. It provides a tool for practitioners, helping them to question basic principles and values, and be clear about what they mean and intend to do. Thus in any situation we should be asking ourselves:

1. Central conditions in working for health
    Am I creating autonomy in my clients, enabling them to direct their own lives?
    Am I respecting the autonomy of my clients whether or not I approve of their chosen direction?
    Am I respecting all people as equal?
    Do I work with people on the basis of needs first?

2. Key principles in working for health
    Am I doing good and avoiding harm?
    Am I telling the truth and keeping promises?

3. Consequences of ways of working for health
    Will my action increase the individual good?
    Will it increase the good of a particular group?
    Will it increase the good of society?
    Will I be acting for the good of myself?

4. External considerations in working for health
    Are there any legal implications?
    Does a professional code of practice suggest a particular course of action?
    Is there a risk attached to the intervention?
    Is the intervention the most effective and efficient action to take?
    How certain is the evidence on which this intervention is based?
    What are the views and wishes of those involved?
    Can I justify my actions in terms of all this evidence?

Questions for further discussion

■ Should we "sell" health?
■ Should there be more legislation to promote health?

Summary

Beneficence, justice and respect for persons and their autonomy are fundamental ethical principles in health promotion. Their application in practice, however, is often problematic. Every situation or potential intervention involves a judgement not only of its possible effectiveness but of its morality – whether it is "right" or "wrong". In this chapter we have defined these key ethical principles and considered how they are manifested in common dilemmas for the health promotion practitioner. The chapter concludes by considering guidelines for ethical practice in health promotion, and their value in steering practitioners and helping them to serve the best interests of clients and populations.

Further reading

Doxiadis S (ed.) (1987) *Ethical Dilemmas in Health Promotion*, Chichester, Wiley.

Contains theoretical chapters which examine the conflict between autonomy and the common good, and then considers practical problems such as the value of health legislation, health economics and paternalism in disease prevention. A final section covers ethical aspects of reproductive medicine, screening programmes and mass communication in health education.

Doxiadis S (ed.) (1990) *Ethics in Health Promotion*, Chichester, Wiley.

Ethical issues in health education are the focus of this book which looks at the ethics of health persuasion and legislation. A final section covers the ethical dilemmas of HIV and AIDS prevention, nutrition education and mental health promotion.

Downie RS, Fyfe C and Tannahill A (1990) *Health Promotion: Models and Values*, Oxford, Oxford Medical Publications.

Chapters 10 and 11 consider the nature of autonomy and justice and the value base for health promotion activities. The book sets out to answer the questions "What is health promotion for and why is it worthwhile?"

Faulder C (1985) *Whose Body Is it?* London, Virago.

A readable study on the controversial issue of informed consent particularly in relation to clinical trials.

Rumbold G (1993) Ethics in Nursing Practice, 2/e, London, Baillière Tindall.

An introduction to ethics and ethical theories and principles. it discusses how these relate to the work of health care workers.

Seedhouse D (1988) *Ethics: The Heart of Health Care*, Chichester, Wiley.

An excellent guide for health promotion practitioners which uses accessible case studies to show how working for health is inextricably bound up with ethics. The Ethical Grid provides a practical framework to be applied in day-to-day work.

References

Beauchamp TL and Childress JF (1989) *Principles of Biomedical Ethics*, Oxford, Oxford University Press.

Campbell AV (1990) "Education or indoctrination? The issue of autonomy in health education", pp. 15–27 in Doxiadis S (ed.) *Ethics in Health Promotion*, Chichester, Wiley.

Craft A (1987) *Mental Handicap and Sexuality: Issues and Perspectives*, Costello.

Doxiadis S (ed.) (1990) *Ethics in Health Promotion*, Chichester, Wiley.

Duncan P (1990) "To screen or not to screen: a question of ethics", *Health Education Journal*, **49**, 120–122.

Ewles L and Simnett I (1992) *Promoting Health*, 2nd edn, Scutari, London.

Gillon R (1990) "Health education: the ambiguity of the medical role", pp. 29–41 in Doxiadis S (ed.) *Ethics in Health Promotion*, Chichester, Wiley.

Frankena WK (1963) *Ethics*, Englewood Cliffs, NJ, Prentice Hall.

Kant I (1909) "On the supposed right to tell lies from benevolent motives", cited in Rumbold (1991). *Ethics in Nursing and Midwifery Practice*, Distance Learning Centre, South Bank University.

Kemm J (1991) "Health education and the problem of knowledge", *Health Promotion International*, **6**, 4 291–269.

Le Fanu (1987) *Eat Your Heart Out*, London, Papermac.

Seedhouse D (1988) *Ethics: The Heart of Health Care*, Chichester, Wiley.

Society of Health Education and Promotion Specialists (1990) *Code of Conduct.* SHE/PS

Tudor Hart J (1971) The Inverse Care Law, *Lancet*, **i**, 405.

UKCC (1992) *Code of Professional Conduct for the Nurse, Midwife and Health Visitor*, London, UKCC.

7

The politics of health promotion

Overview

Politics and health promotion are often thought of as separate activities. In this chapter we shall consider how these two areas overlap, and will argue that health promotion cannot be considered in isolation from the broader arena of politics. We shall outline how politics may be theorized and provide a framework for considering different political ideologies. The proposition that health promotion is an inherently political activity will then be examined in relation to three areas: the structure, methods and content of health promotion activity. Finally, we shall discuss the dilemmas facing the self-confessed radical practitioner, who is at the stage of recognizing that their health promotion work has political implications, and wishes to make positive use of this fact.

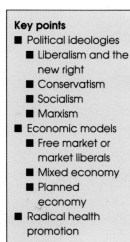

Key points
- Political ideologies
  - Liberalism and the new right
  - Conservatism
  - Socialism
  - Marxism
- Economic models
  - Free market or market liberals
  - Mixed economy
  - Planned economy
- Radical health promotion

What is politics?

Politics is most often thought of as relating to party politics but we shall use a broader definition of the term in this chapter. Politics may be defined as the study of the distribution and effects of power in society. Power itself may be defined in different ways. Power includes not only material or physical resources, but also psychological and cultural aspects, which may be equally effective in limiting or channelling people.

No one is totally devoid of power and no one is all powerful. But within a highly stratified society, such as Britain, different groups of people typically will possess different amounts of power. Although we live in a democratic society with one person one vote, power is unequally distributed. Gender, race, social class, wealth and disability structure power relationships between groups of people, and this has effects on health, as discussed in Chapter 2. Structural factors such as class and gender affect power relationships in an institutionalized and patterned manner. In general, people in the lower social classes and women have less control over their own lives, and the lives of others compared to men in higher social classes. But it is impossible to predict the power relationships between people. This is due both to the complexity of the inter-relationship between different factors, and also to personal power or charisma which exists in the relationships between actual people. People in subordinate positions may have the opportunity and skills to exercise a greater degree of power or influence than could be anticipated. Hence the well-known phenomenon of the receptionist or secretary who is said to "run the office".

One of the arenas in which power relationships are manifest is social policy, which may be defined as planned Government activities designed to maintain, integrate and regulate society. This includes both welfare and economic policies, ranging from national legislation to local policy developments within local authorities. Different political positions give rise to certain types of policy interventions. Analysts have identified many different frameworks (George and Wilding, 1976; Lee and Raban, 1988; Williams, 1989; Bunton, 1992). In general, ideological positions are identified along a spectrum ranging from those advocating a free market economy with minimal state intervention to those advocating a planned economy with maximum state intervention. Conservatives or socialists who advocate a mixed economy and a welfare state occupy the middle of the spectrum.

Different beliefs and values underly these different perspectives. On the right of the political spectrum there is a belief in individual self-determination and an antipathy to Government intervention which not only restricts freedom, but also inhibits enterprise. Conservatism sees inequality as inevitable but advocates a paternalistic state which safeguards the most vulnerable. Socialism is based on a belief in equality and fellowship, or a sense of responsibility for others. The Government has a distinct role to play in redistributing material resources and promoting a sense of community. Marxism embraces the values of equality, collective responsibility and freedom from want. To achieve these goals requires revolutionary change and the transformation of the capitalist state to a Marxist state. The Marxist state has a key role in planning the economy to meet needs. Table 7.1 below gives an illustration of this.

It has been argued that these accounts focus on the effects of policy on class inequalities. Until these accounts consider the impact of policy on gender and racial inequalities, they will remain partial and inadequate (Williams, 1989).

Following the Second World War, British policy favoured a middle point in the spectrum. All political parties were united by a consensus that the Welfare State was a desirable goal and that a certain amount of state intervention was necessary. From a "one nation" Tory point of view, state intervention was necessary to curb the worst excesses of capitalism, which left some people without

Table 7.1 A typology of welfare ideologies.

	(Political Right)			(Political left)
Political ideology	Liberalism/new right	Conservatism	Fabian socialism	Marxism
Role of state	Anti-collectivist	Reluctant collectivists	Collectivist	Collectivist
View of economy	Free market Market liberals	Mixed economy	Mixed economy	Planned economy
View of society	Inequalities in wealth are inevitable Market forces ensure people's needs are met in a satisfactory manner	Inequality is inevitable but there should be equality of opportunity The State's role is to provide for the vulnerable and needy, but individual freedom of choice must be protected	Equality of opportunity, economic and political freedom is safe-guarded by the State The State should enable individual self-fulfilment and social justice through redistribution	Present class society characterized by class conflict will be superseded by socialism characterized by "from each according to their ability; to each according to their need."
View of health care	Individual responsibility and freedom of choice Needs are best met through the free market Consumerism	Paternalistic State should provide a safety net of health care provision, alongside individual responsibility	Universal and free State provision to promote social cohesion and redistribution plus individual provision if desired	Universal and free State provision
Core values	Individualism Freedom Choice Competition	Individualism Freedom Responsibility Authority	Equality Collective responsibility Humanitarianism Social harmony Social justice	Equality Collective responsibility Freedom from material want

means of support. For example, if capitalist recession leads to mass unemployment, it is legitimate to intervene to protect the unemployed from destitution. Without this intervention, the system becomes unstable. From a socialist perspective, the Welfare State is a means of gradually reforming the State from within. The Welfare State is a means of redistributing wealth, and incremental reforms are capable of transforming the State from an instrument of capitalism to an instrument of socialism.

This consensus was disrupted by the economic recession and fiscal crisis of the mid-1970s. The burgeoning costs of welfare, triggered by the changing demographic structure of the population and mass unemployment, gave rise to Government concern, and set the scene for the ascendency of a new political ideology. The new right or Thatcherism became the dominant ideology in the 1980s. The new right is characterized by a more *laissez-faire* attitude favouring no State intervention in the economy. It is argued that the State needs to retreat from its commitment to welfare. The Welfare State is seen as having undesirable effects, such as raising the level of expectations beyond what can be provided. Universal provision for all denies individual choices and is an ineffective means of meeting needs. In addition, the Welfare State transforms people into dependents and saps their independence. The free market is seen as a more desirable means for meeting welfare needs. The free market protects individual choice, and will lead to a more rational provision of goods and services, as only those things for which there is a demonstrable need will be produced. Competition will reduce wastage and inefficiencies in the system.

The new right combines this economic liberal or *laissez-faire* attitude with a conservative authoritarianism which prioritizes the need for strong moral values and authority invested in the power of the State. This combination means that, at the same time as Government is retreating from economic intervention, it is engaged in extending State power over the everyday lives of the population.

? **Consider the social policy interventions referred to in these newspaper headlines: Do such measures increase individual choice? Do such measures represent a more effective use of resources?**

- Patients become consumers with the right to choose
- Hospitals forced into competitive tendering to provide services for health districts
- New moves to force absent fathers to provide for their children
- Government accused of phone bugging
- Privatization of water and railways to go ahead
- GP fundholders shop around for the best deal for their patients
- Workfair proposals to make unemployed work to earn their benefits
- Stop the nanny state and the do-gooders from taking over our lives
- Minister calls for parents to be responsible for crimes committed by their children
- Single parents to blame for the rise in juvenile crime
- Social workers remove children from alleged satanic abuse.

The political context affects all areas of Government policy including health. The central proposition of this chapter is that health promotion takes place in the policy arena and is, therefore, inescapably, a political activity. The next sections will examine the evidence for this proposition, looking first at the structure and organization of health promotion, then at its methods, and finally at the content of health promotion.

The politics of health promotion structures and organization

Health promotion has enjoyed varying levels of Government support throughout the 20th century. In most recent times, health education and promotion was enthusiastically supported in the mid-1970s and again in the beginning of the 1990s. The Department of Health and Social Security (DHSS) report, *Prevention and Health: Everybody's Business*, was published in 1976, and was followed by other reports which examined health promotion in relation to specific topics such as heart disease and alcohol (DHSS, 1981a, 1981b). It has been argued that the timing of these reports was no coincidence. With the economic crisis of the mid-1970s, health promotion came to be viewed as a means of cost cutting. If people could be prevented from becoming ill, health service costs could be reduced and economic productivity increased. It is interesting to note that the current resurgence of interest in health promotion and the publication of *The Health of the Nation* in 1992 have also occurred at a time of economic recession.

Whilst health promotion is seen as "everybody's business", certain groups and organizational settings have been identified as the base for health promotion specialists. In Britain, the National Health Service (NHS) has come to be regarded as the natural home for health promotion. The division of responsibilities in the 1970s, which separated environmental health (located in local authorities) from community health and health promotion (located in the NHS) has had important repercussions. Health promotion has become subordinated to health care provision and the medical model dominates amongst health professionals. The siting of health promotion within the NHS has made it more difficult to influence other factors which affect health, such as housing, education, transport and leisure facilities.

Any account of the current structure and organization of health promotion services in Britain is in danger of becoming out of date in the very near future. However, a brief outline is useful in order to locate the development of health promotion within the framework of political ideologies given earlier.

The responsibility for health promotion is divided between different groups within the NHS and, to a lesser extent, groups outside the NHS. Within the NHS there is a national lead body, the Health Education Authority (HEA), which is responsible for research and the development and dissemination of national programmes. In 1987 the HEA was constituted as a special health authority, directly responsible to the Department of Health, replacing the Health Education Council quango (quasi-autonomous non-governmental organization).

It has been argued that this change brought the HEA under more Governmental control, and that its former independence was compromised (Brindle 1989).

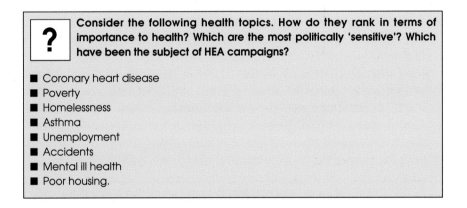

? Consider the following health topics. How do they rank in terms of importance to health? Which are the most politically 'sensitive'? Which have been the subject of HEA campaigns?

- Coronary heart disease
- Poverty
- Homelessness
- Asthma
- Unemployment
- Accidents
- Mental ill health
- Poor housing.

The NHS and Community Care Act of 1991 divided health authorities into purchasers and providers (Department of Health, 1991). The purchasing authority has responsibility for determining health needs and commissioning appropriate services from provider services for its population.

Health promotion may be part of the purchasing authority, or part of the provider services, or may be divided between the two. Different health authorities around the country have opted for different arrangements.

The implications of this are far reaching. If health promotion is to be proactive and concern itself with the assessment of need, it should be located in the purchasing authority. If it is to be a provider service, there is the possibility that health promotion services within the NHS will have to bid amongst competing services from the private sector (such as occupational health services, drug company education departments or freelance trainers) to win contracts. As a provider service, health promotion would be less able to exercise autonomy in relation to its own development. Bidding for contracts entails target setting, which emphasizes those aspects of health promotion which can be quantified, such as the number of training sessions held. More innovative, qualitative and long-term types of health promotion, such as community development, are unlikely to figure in contract specifications.

In addition to these changes in the structure of health authorities, the new Government funding arrangements for GPs have clearly signalled the intention that primary care should take a lead role for health promotion. The new GP contract has three levels of payment linked to the degree of health promotion activities undertaken within the practice – the new banding arrangements. The Family Health Services Authority (FHSA), which administers payments to GPs, dentists, opticians and pharmacists, has been given the task of administering and monitoring the new banding payments. Band 1, with the lowest payment, requires GPs to adopt a programme to reduce smoking. The middle, Band 2, requires a programme to minimize mortality and morbidity from hypertension, coronary heart disease (CHD) or stroke. The top, Band 3, requires a health promotion programme offering a full range of primary prevention of CHD and stroke. There are separate payments for organizing a chronic disease management programme for either asthma and/or diabetes (General Medical Services Committee, 1993).

 Consider these developments in health promotion policy in the context of health promotion models, discussed in Chapter 5.
What kind of model(s) of health promotion do these developments imply?

The approaches favoured by these arrangements are medical preventive and those which focus on individual lifestyles. The new GP payment structures send a clear message about what is considered appropriate and effective health promotion. The medical preventive model is evident in the prioritizing of action on CHD and stroke, and, to a lesser extent, asthma and diabetes. Health promotion is seen as a means to prevent morbidity and mortality from specified diseases. Creating a database of the practice population, including health surveillance information, is an integral feature of the banding payments. Lifestyles are also prioritized. It is envisaged that health surveillance will identify personal risk factors for CHD and other diseases. Lifestyle interventions by primary health care staff are seen as the means to achieve health goals. So policy developments in health promotion have the effect of legitimizing certain approaches to health promotion and ignoring others.

Changes in other organizations have contributed to this retrenchment of health promotion within the NHS. New duties imposed on environmental health departments by the European Community have not been matched by an increase in funding or staffing. This has led to several local authorities disbanding health promotion departments, as the new statutory duties must take precedence. Local management in schools has led to a reduction in the budget and responsibilities of Local Education Authorities. One response has been the disbanding of the former special advisors in health education, who provided a co-ordinating and training function to support health education in schools.

The overall effect of these policy and organizational changes has been to strengthen the medical and lifestyles approaches to health promotion. There has been an accompanying loss of diversity in practice. Health promotion activity is being more narrowly interpreted, and more tightly controlled, than in previous years. Whilst it could be argued that greater accountability is desirable, the opportunities for democratic accountability have been reduced. The new managerialism in the NHS has strengthened managerial power at the expense of both professional and lay power. Health authority membership has been reduced, with the loss of elected representatives. The future of the lay forum within the NHS, the community health councils, is uncertain. Yet at the same time, the justification for such changes is said to be to extend patient choice.

The combination of free-market economics (money following patients who become consumers of services) with authoritarianism (top-down approaches of medical and lifestyles health promotion) fits into the new right political ideology. It is apparent that health promotion activities are structured by the prevailing policy framework. Certain health promotion strategies become the preferred types of intervention and mainstream Government funding for these strategies becomes available. Alternative and oppositional health promotion strategies such as community development survive but in a precarious environment characterized by short-term funding.

The politics of health promotion methods

The methods used in health promotion are often viewed as a technical choice. Health promotion specialists are seen as possessing the expertise to decide what methods will prove most effective given the circumstances. However, we shall argue that methods imply political perspectives, and that the choice of which methods to use is not a politically neutral decision.

Health promotion has at its disposal a large repertoire of methods. These are discussed in greater detail in Chapter 13.

Beattie's typology of health promotion classifies health promotion models according to two dimensions, the focus of intervention and the mode of intervention (Beattie, 1991). Health promotion methods may be similarly classified. Figure 7.1 below gives an illustration of this.

Figure 7.1 is not an exhaustive list of the repertoire of health promotion methods but it does indicate the range of methods used in health promotion. We shall consider each cell in turn, identifying the methods used and tracing their political implications.

The individual authoritarian

The individual authoritarian cell would include a variety of methods including giving advice, education and behaviour-change interventions such as lifestyle clinics. Mass media is also included as, although it is a means of mass communication, it addresses people as individuals. For example, "No Smoking Day" addresses individual smokers and their desire to quit, the AIDS campaign focused on the individual responsibility to practise safer sex, and "Look After Your Heart" emphasizes the individual responsibility to reduce personal risk factors such as eating too much saturated fat or lack of exercise. Mass media campaigns were included as a central strategy in all these programmes.

Figure 7.1 Health promotion methods using Beattie's (1991) typology of health promotion.

MODE OF INTERVENTION
Authoritarian

Advice
Education
Behaviour change
interventions
Mass media campaigns

Legislation
Policy-making and
implementation
Health surveillance

Individual

Collective

Focus of
intervention

Counselling
Education
Group work

Lobbying
Action research
Skills sharing and training
Group work
Community development

Negotiated

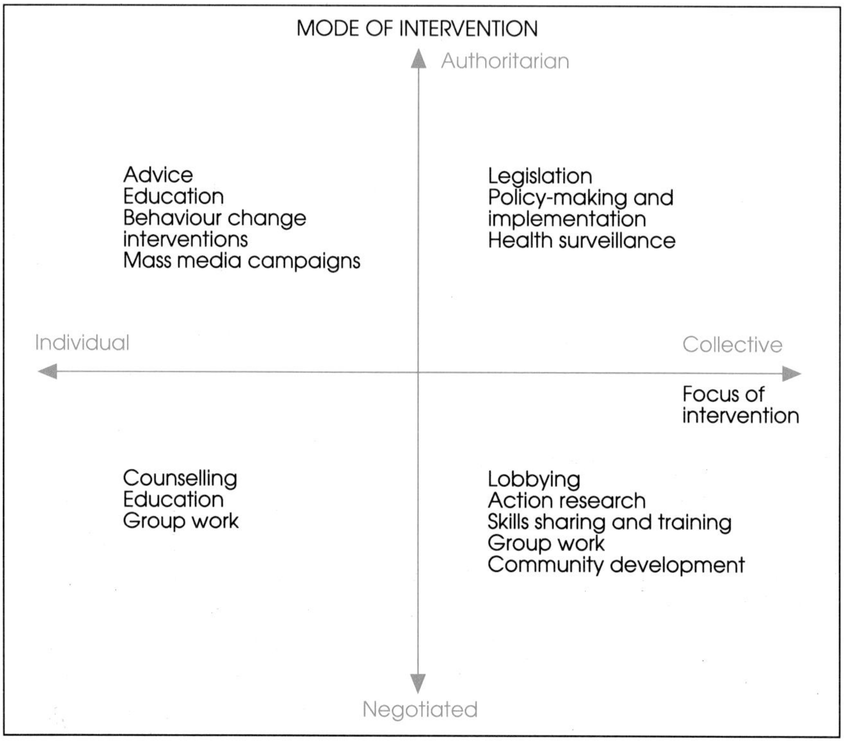

Methods focused on the individual send a clear message about individual responsibility for health. Such methods rely on the belief that the individual can make significant changes in their lifestyle or environment. The focus on the individual also implies that all individuals have equal resources and means of complying with health promotion messages. This may be viewed as ineffective, or incorrect, and there has been much criticism of these methods in these terms, as 'victim-blaming' and misconceived (Naidoo 1986). However, such a viewpoint is also politically inspired, which may go some way to explaining its endurance in the face of professional criticism.

By ignoring structural factors which affect the life chances and perceptions of different groups of people, the fact that people's personal identity is bound up with their membership of such groups is obscured.

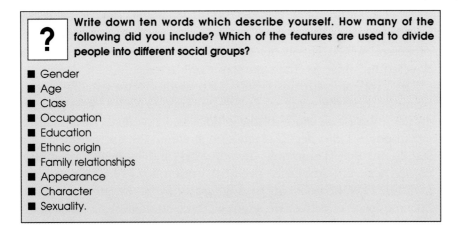

? Write down ten words which describe yourself. How many of the following did you include? Which of the features are used to divide people into different social groups?

- Gender
- Age
- Class
- Occupation
- Education
- Ethnic origin
- Family relationships
- Appearance
- Character
- Sexuality.

The individual is presented in a social vacuum, as a neutral phenomenon, which assures everyone of equal opportunities. In fact, individualism is firmly entrenched in liberalism and the new right. The notion of individual free choice is a central tenet of both the free-market economy and liberal political ideology. By contrast, socialism and Marxism prioritize the collectivity, people united by circumstances into groups with opposing interests.

The individual negotiated

The individual negotiated cell includes methods such as counselling, education and groupwork. These methods envisage a different, and more equal, relationship between the health promoter and the client than those derived from the individual authoritarian cell. The health promotion intervention is to be negotiated between both parties, taking into account people's beliefs, attitudes and knowledge. The client is an active partner in

What criticisms can be offered of this approach in terms of promoting the nation's health?

the process and the end goal is enhanced client autonomy. For these reasons, many health promoters feel more comfortable using these methods.

It may be argued that individually negotiated methods are most used and valued by the relatively privileged and healthy sections of society. Those with the greatest need are least likely to be able to access this kind of health promotion intervention. It may also be argued that such an intervention is not what is required when there are basic health needs going unmet.

The collective negotiated

Methods which focus on the collectivity are more likely to be allied to socialist or Marxist political ideologies. This is certainly true of the collective negotiated methods of health promotion, which seek to redistribute power by empowering disadvantaged groups through such means as action research, skills sharing and training, and lobbying. The emphasis here is on understanding the processes which shape health outcomes, and assisting people to develop the skills to challenge these processes.

The problem with this is that such methods are usually seen as being beyond the remit of health workers. O'Neill (1989) presents an interesting case study of the pitfalls and potentials of attempting to tap politics into health promotion strategies. Starting from a clear standpoint that "community health work and its health promotion component are primarily political undertakings" (O'Neill, 1989, p. 228), O'Neill goes on to suggest how health promoters can become more effective. He suggests three strategies:

■ Action research in which researchers and researched are equal partners
■ Tapping political considerations into programme planning
■ Providing training to develop the political skills of health promoters.

The collective authoritarian

The collective authoritarian methods of working may be located in either the Marxist or new right political ideologies, depending on the underlying values and purposes of such methods. For Marxists, the collectivity is structured into opposing classes by social stratification variables. Appropriate action uses methods such as the active redistribution of power in favour of the disadvantaged, which is also advocated by socialist groups. Examples of this are proposals to improve housing, increase maternity benefits, or to provide free school meals. All of these measures are supported by research as effective means of improving health and reducing health inequalities (Townsend *et al.*, 1988).

On the other hand, the new right represents the collectivity as the sum total of many individuals, each with different and competing interests. Appropriate intervention is then designed to protect individual rights, which may only be superseded to protect the common good or the wider body politic. For example, immunization is an imposition on individual freedom but may be supported because it helps protect the health of the whole community. The tension between individual freedom and community well-being may explain why immunization remains voluntary in Britain, whereas in other countries, including the USA, child immunization is a prerequisite of school enrolment. Another example is health surveillance of the general population. Although this does not necessarily benefit the individual, it may be advocated as providing the necessary information on which to base strategies to improve the health of everyone. Health surveillance is a central strategy in the Government's health promotion policy, and is a major component of both *Health of the Nation* and the new GP contract.

This discussion has presented the view that the methods chosen to promote health are not politically neutral. Certain methods fit into, maintain and reproduce the ideological assumptions of certain political perspectives. However, it is important not to overstate this view. Methods and ideology are not deterministically linked in a cause and effect manner. A variety of methods across all four cells may be used by health workers who espouse a particular political viewpoint. There may be convincing reasons for adopting an eclectic methodology to promote health. But it is a fallacy to assume that methods are a technically neutral aspect of the health promoter's activity.

The politics of health promotion content

The previous sections have examined the view that the structure, organization and methods used in health promotion have a political dimension. It is sometimes argued that, although the process of promoting health is a political activity, the content of health promotion is neutral. Our position is that health promotion content is inevitably political. The framing of suitable agendas and the construction of what information is relevant are not value neutral activities. On the contrary, they imply certain political values.

Perhaps the clearest example of the political nature of health promotion content is the ongoing debate surrounding inequalities in health. Whilst there is a wealth of research evidence linking poverty and disadvantage with ill health (Townsend *et al.*, 1988; Association of CHCs, 1991), the Government has consistently refused to recognize this.

What are the health issues which should be addressed by the health promoter?

"Health is a state of complete physical, mental and social well-being, and not merely the absence of disease or infirmity" (WHO, 1948)

"Health for all implies *equity*. This means that the present inequalities in health between countries and within countries should be reduced as far as possible" (WHO, 1985, p. 5, original emphasis)

"No-one is immortal, but in many cases the onset of illness can be prevented or delayed. When illness strikes, treatment aimed at cure or rehabilitation will continue to be of prime importance. But it is of equal importance to promote good health and well-being, thus preventing illness in the first place" (Department of Health, 1992, p. 14).

 In 1980 the Government released a limited number of copies of the Black Report on health inequalities over a bank holiday weekend. The recommendations of the Black Report included Government investment and spending on housing, pre-school child care, child benefits, maternity grants and free school meals in order to reduce inequalities in health.

How could you explain Government action in the light of what the report contained?

Accepting the evidence, and the desirability of a healthy population, would lead the Government to adopt a policy of active intervention to reduce inequalities (similar to the socialist position in Table 7.1). By denying the evidence, Government can justify a non-interventionist policy and argue that the free market is the best means of meeting health needs. The recent *Health of the Nation* document does not even acknowledge health inequalities as an issue, referring only to "variations in health status between different socio-economic groups within the population" (Department of Health, 1992, p.121).

There is as much academic consensus on the issue of health inequalities as on any other health topic. In other words, there is an overwhelming but less than total agreement that poverty and disadvantage are responsible for poor health outcomes. Yet in official circles this evidence is consistently disregarded, from what can only be political motives.

To recap, our argument so far has been that:

■ The dominant view of health promotion is about preventing illness, with the focus on specific diseases, risk factors and target groups. This is apparent in the *Health of the Nation* document and local plans which have been produced to meet the targets set.

■ This view of health, derived from the medical model, is narrow, and risk factors are personal lifestyle factors.

■ The emphasis is on education and persuasion to get people to voluntarily adopt healthier lifestyles.

■ Legislation or coercion to achieve better health is not acceptable, as it curtails individual freedom.

■ It is apparent that this view of health and health promotion fits into the new right perspective, with its mix of authoritarianism (doctors know best about health as well as illness) and *laissez-faire* economics (people have the right to choose healthy or unhealthy products in an unregulated marketplace).

> **?** The following are a list of health promotion interventions. List them according to the political perspective (new right/liberal, conservative, socialist, Marxist) with which they are most associated.
>
> ■ Health surveillance of those over 75
> ■ Legislation to ban cigarette advertising
> ■ A voluntary agreement with food companies to label the fat content of products
> ■ Price fixing to make healthier foods relatively cheaper
> ■ Universal free school meals providing one third of nutritional requirements for children
> ■ Two-tier health care system, separated into universal basic provision for those who cannot afford private care, and private provision for those who can
> ■ Mass education campaign to reduce personal lifestyle risk factors for CHD
> ■ Housing programme to provide subsidized housing meeting minimum health and safety requirements for those unable to buy their own homes
> ■ Benefits system to provide a "safety net" income for those without means of support.

The debate about what is a legitimate health concern is continuing. Whilst there is little disagreement that major causes of disability and premature death, such as the five key topics identified in the *Health of the Nation* (CHD, cancers, accidents, mental health and sexual health) deserve attention, there is disagreement concerning other known causes of ill health, such as poor housing, unemployment or low income. The Government has yet to acknowledge these factors as health issues, and is not willing to intervene and address these issues on health grounds. Even with lifestyle risk factors, such as diet and smoking, the preferred policy is to advise and educate individuals, but not to intervene in the economic sphere which shapes consumer choices. This is the rationale for the Government's much-criticized refusal to ban cigarette advertising, whilst simultaneously funding health promotion campaigns such as "No Smoking Day".

If a health topic is constructed so that it mixes with other topics of central concern, such as maintaining law and order, it is more likely to receive recognition and funding.

The medical model of health is often welcomed by health professionals because it provides them with a clear role, and recognizes and rewards their expertise. On an everyday level, health workers want to prevent ill health, but find their activities curtailed by their professional training and contractual obligations. They may embrace the medical model of health because this provides them with a way of extending their role from care and cure to prevention.

Ilegal drug use and drink driving have both been the subject of major Government mass-media campaigns in the last decade. Why do you think these particular topics have been chosen?

> **?** **A survey of Bath Health Authority residents in 1986 included the following amongst identified health priorities.**
>
> Which of these topics do you feel you could legitimately address as part of your professional role?
>
> - The threat of nuclear war
> - Lack of suitable housing
> - Having a secure job
> - Having enough money to live on
> - Stress
> - Smoking, alcohol and illegal drugs
> - Being able to keep warm in winter
> - Accidents
> - Noise
> - A good sex life
>
> Source: Farrell, 1986.

Health education or giving information is often viewed as a neutral activity, with no political undertones. Scientific research is said to have identified certain risk factors for disease, and the health worker's role is to impart this knowledge to clients in an accessible way. This view of scientific neutrality has been criticized by social scientists (Kuhn, 1962; Chalmers, 1982), who point out that science is a social activity like any other, subject to similar constraints. Health-related research does not take place in ivory towers. Researchers have to bid for funds, and provide findings which are acceptable to funders and the academic community.

>
>
> - In 1989 Margaret Thatcher vetoed a proposed survey of people's sexual habits as part of the HEA's HIV/AIDS prevention strategy because she thought it intruded too much in people's personal affairs.
> - Many health promotion researchers have accepted money from the tobacco industry's Health Promotion Trust in order to carry out their research.
> - The British Nutrition Foundation, which funds research into diet and health, is sponsored by major food producers.
> - Researchers in Scotland were unable to gain funding to continue their research into the links between unemployment and health, and poor housing and health.

The process of research is therefore not immune to political considerations. What evidence filters through to the general public as the scientific consensus on health topics is also the result of political processes. The very idea of scientific consensus in social science is debatable. There is no issue where there is 100% agreement of the 'scientific facts'. There are still scientists (albeit funded by the tobacco industry) who claim the causal link between cigarette smoking and lung cancer is unproven (FOREST, 1981) and who contest the evidence that passive smoking is a health hazard (Huber, *et al.*, 1993). And there are researchers who dispute the links between saturated fats and CHD (Le Fanu, 1987). However, the HEA's statements about its role in health education appear to imply that information is not problematic, and that there is complete agreement about what the health messages should be:

"[The HEA's mission is] to help the people of England to become more knowledgeable, better motivated, and more able to acquire and maintain good health" (HEA, 1993, p.2).

Assuming that a consensus exists makes it easier to justify an authoritarian or expert-dominated approach to health education.

Radical health promotion

We have seen how most mainstream health promotion arises from and reinforces new right political values and beliefs. This will be relatively unproblematic for health promoters who identify with these beliefs, because their professional duties will be in accordance (more or less) with their personal values. But for health promoters who espouse a different political philosophy, it is likely that their professional role will at times come into conflict with their political beliefs and values. This section will explore these dilemmas and suggest some responses.

"Radical health promotion" has been coined as the term to identify health promotion which seeks to promote the political values of the broad left. Tones' model (Figure 7.2) (cited in Jones, 1985) identifies different aspects of radical health education.

Aggleton and Whitty (1986) view radical health promotion as not merely critical of the *status quo* but oppositional, that is, it seeks to transform social conditions in order to promote health. They suggest that the best means of doing this is to develop broad alliances around popular issues. An example of this would be the campaigns to save the NHS during the period of reform in the 1980s.

The development of a critical understanding around health issues, in order to identify options and priorities, is also a primary task for health promoters. This requires an open, sharing and egalitarian relationship between health promoters and the public. Aggleton and Whitty state that moves to professionalize health promotion seek to increase the social distance between health promoters and clients, and are therefore incompatible with radical practice.

This interpretation of radical health promotion may appear daunting to individual health promoters. How can the demands of the job be reconciled with such activities? There are only so many hours in a day, and statutory duties, caseloads, and contractual

Research into cervical cancer has identified several risk factors. These include:

- Heterosexuality
- Number of sexual partners
- Age of first sexual intercourse
- Non-barrier means of contraception
- Male partners working in dusty occupations (such as builders).

The first and last of these risk factors have received little attention. Government health education programmes have stressed the second and third factors. Is this a political agenda? Source: Robinson, 1983.

Figure 7.2 Tones' model of radical health education (source: Tones, cited in Jones, 1985).

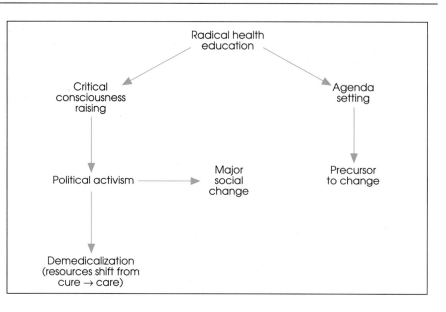

obligations may leave little or no leeway for developing such activities. The following activity is designed to help radical health promoters identify where they could make changes in their practice.

 The following are suggestions for developing radical health promotion practice. How many do you think are feasible for you? Be clear and honest about your own political standpoint.

■ Develop an equal relationship with clients, where beliefs and values are respected, and information shared
■ Try to ensure real community involvement in policies and decision-making
■ Try to address health as a collective issue, making explicit the facts about health inequalities and supporting collective action around health issues
■ Vet the health education materials you use to ensure they do not reproduce stereotypes or assumptions about gender, class, race, disability, age or sexuality
■ Develop a support network with like-minded health workers, where perspectives can be shared and issues discussed
■ Be honest to yourself and others about the limitations of your work role.
Adapted from Adams and Slavin, 1985.

Conclusion

There is often resistance to the idea that health promotion is a political activity. Accepting the premise that politics is involved in health promotion may be experienced as muddying the waters, for it transforms a situation of relative certainty to one of uncertainty. It is no longer sufficient to rely on professional training to ensure effective health promotion. A whole range of different considerations needs to be taken into account, some of which threaten and call into question the whole notion of professional expertise.

However uncomfortable the process may be, an awareness of the political nature of health promotion is vital to its effectiveness (O'Neill, 1989). Accepting the *status quo* is not an apolitical position but a deeply political one. What exists is not inevitable, but the result of complex forces and historical processes. Things might be otherwise. Health promotion is centrally concerned with a vision of better health for all. This vision may be informed by scientific knowledge and technical know-how, but its overall shape is determined by personal values and beliefs. Part of the health promoter's task is to uncover and hold up to scrutiny their values and beliefs. It is hoped that this chapter and Chapter 6 on ethics will help health promoters in this task.

Questions for further discussion

■ To what extent may health promotion be said to be a political activity?
■ How could an understanding of politics help the health promoter develop more effective practice?

Summary

This chapter has examined the political implications of health promotion structure, organization, methods and content. The central proposition is that health promotion is a political activity, and that to attempt to deny this lessens one's understanding and the possibility of effective action. It has been demonstrated that mainstream health promotion activity is predicated on certain political values associated with the new right. These political values combine an authoritarian attitude which reinforces the power of the experts with a *laissez-faire* or non-interventionist attitude to the economy, and a belief that people's needs are best met in a free-market economy. For health workers who espouse these political beliefs, there will be little or no conflict between their work role and their values. However, for health workers who hold differing political beliefs, there may well be tension between what they are able to do as part of their work role, and what they would like to be doing. For these people, it is important to identify how they can adapt or modify their work role to enable their work to be more congruent with their beliefs and values.

Further reading

Bunton R (1992) "Health promotion as social policy", in Bunton R and Macdonald G (eds) *Health Promotion: Disciplines and Diversity*, London, Routledge.

A useful discussion of health promotion as social policy, identifying different political perspectives. It uses alcohol policies as a case study to explore the issues.

O'Neill M (1989) "The political dimension of health promotion work", in Martin CJ and McQueen DV (eds) *Readings for a New Public Health*, Edinburgh, Edinburgh University Press.

A chapter which explores how political awareness and skills, which are needed to enhance health promotion work, may be tapped into health workers' training. Obstacles to this process are identified and discussed. The case study used is Canadian.

References

Adams L and Slavin H (1985) "Checklist for personal action", *Radical Health Promotion*, **2**, 47.

Aggleton P and Whitty G (1986) "Components of a radical health education practice", *Radical Health Promotion*, **4**, 24–28.

Association of Community Health Councils in England and Wales (1991) *Health and Wealth.*

Beattie A (1991) "Knowledge and control in health promotion: a test case for social policy and social theory", in J Gabe, M Calnan and M Bury (eds) *The Sociology of the Health Service*, pp. 162–201, London, Routledge.

Brindle D (1989) "Controversy clouds future", *The Guardian*, 6/12/89.

Bunton R (1992) "Health promotion as social policy", in Bunton R and Macdonald G (eds) *Health Promotion: Disciplines and Diversity*, pp. 129–152, London, Routledge.

Chalmers A (1982) *What is This Thing Called Science?* Milton Keynes, Open University Press.

Department of Health (1991) *NHS and Community Care Act*, London, HMSO.

Department of Health (1992) *The Health of the Nation*, London, HMSO.

Department of Health and Social Security (1976) *Prevention and Health: Everybody's Business*, London, HMSO.

Department of Health and Social Security (1981a) *Prevention and Health: Avoiding heart attacks*, London, HMSO.

Department of Health and Social Security (1981b) *Drinking Sensibly*, London, HMSO.

Farrell E (1986) *Marketing Research for Local Health Promotion*, HEC Research Report 7, London, Health Education Council.

Freedom Organisation for the Right to Enjoy Smoking Tobacco (FOREST) (1981) *Newsletter* No. 4.

General Medical Services Committee (1993) *The New Health Promotion Package*, London, British Medical Association.

George P and Wilding P (1976) *Ideology and Social Welfare*, London, Routledge and Kegan Paul.

Health Education Authority (1993) *Strategy 1993–1998*, London, HEA.

Huber GL, Brockie RE and Mahajan VK (1993) *Passive Smoking: How Great a Hazard?* FOREST Information Sheet No. 5.

Jones L (1985) "On being radical", *Radical Health Promotion*, **2**, 3–5.

Kuhn T (1962) *The Structure of Scientific Revolutions*, Chicago, University of Chicago Press.

Lee P and Raban C (1988) "Welfare and ideology", in Loney M *et al.* (eds) *Social Policy and Social Welfare*, pp. 18–32, Milton Keynes, Open University Press.

Le Fanu J (1987) *Eat Your Heart Out*, London, Papermac.

Naidoo J (1986) "Limits to individualism", in Rodmell S and Watt A (eds) *The Politics of Health Education*, pp. 17–37, London, Routledge and Kegan Paul.

O'Neill M (1989) "The political dimension of health promotion work", in Martin CJ and McQueen DV (eds) *Readings for a New Public Health*, pp. 222–234, Edinburgh, Edinburgh University Press.

Robinson J (1983) "Cervical cancer: occupational risks", *The Lancet*, **2**, 1496-1497.

Townsend P, Davidson N and Whitehead M (1988) *Inequalities in Health: The Black Report and the Health Divide*, Harmondsworth, Penguin.

Williams F (1989) *Social Policy: A Critical Introduction*, Cambridge, Polity Press.

World Health Organisation (1948) *Constitution*, Geneva, WHO.

World Health Organisation (1985) *Targets for Health for All*, Copenhagen, WHO Regional Office for Europe.

Healthy alliances – working together

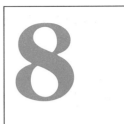

Overview

In Chapter 4 we explored the shift in health promotion towards a broad view of health encompassing social and environmental factors. Improving health cannot, therefore, be the sole responsibility of the National Health Service (NHS). A wide range of organizations and agencies influences the health of the population including education, environmental health, industry and commerce, social welfare and voluntary groups. The national strategy to focus on health gain requires these agencies to be brought into partnership with communities to develop a common agenda for promoting positive health. The World Health Organisation calls this process **intersectoral collaboration**. The Government White Paper *The Health of the Nation* calls it establishing healthy alliances.

> **Key points**
> ■ Definitions of "healthy alliances" and ways of working together
> ■ Characteristics of successful teams
> ■ Main stakeholders in the promotion of health

Definitions

There are many different terms that are used to describe the ways that people work together to promote health. Although these are often used interchangeably it is possible to distinguish between them:

■ **Multi-agency** refers to organizations that belong to the same sector such as health, social services, or education who are all statutory providers of public services.

■ **Intersectoral** goes beyond any one sector and may include public, private (business and commerce) and voluntary groups.

■ **Inter- or multi-disciplinary working** is sometimes used to describe joint working of people with different roles or functions within the same organization or across sectors.

■ **Joint planning**. Organizations within or across sectors agree objectives, and meet regularly to develop and implement a joint plan.

■ **Teams.** Teams usually have a common task and are made up of people chosen because they have relevant expertise. They may be multidisciplinary such as a Primary Health Care Team or a team who work in the same organization or they may be inter-agency such as an HIV Team or Child Protection Team.

> **?**   **Think of a task you currently undertake which involves working with others in a team or where you share care with someone else.**
>
> ■ Who is or should be members of the team and why have they been chosen?
> ■ Does everyone understand their role and those of the other members?
> ■ Is everyone committed to the task and the methods to be used?
> ■ How frequently do you meet to plan and review the task?
> ■ Does the team discuss its own progress and development?
> ■ Who leads the team and why?
>
> You may not work in an established team or project but nevertheless work with other people in promoting health.
> ■ Are there any ways you could develop stronger links with other staff in your own or other organizations?
> ■ Are there opportunities for joint planning, target setting or joint aims and objectives?

Background

Collaboration in health promotion received a major impetus with the publication of the health strategy *Health of the Nation* (Department of Health, 1992). This represented the first attempt to propose a national strategy for health, and acknowledged that this would require the active participation of a wide range of departments and agencies at national and local level. The Health of the Nation handbook defines healthy alliances as "in effect, a partnership of individuals and organizations formed to enable people to increase their influence over the factors that affect their health and well-being – physically, mentally, socially, and environmentally" (Department of Health, 1993). Although the strategy may appear to be one for the NHS rather than for health, and be criticized for its focus on disease rather than on social factors producing ill health, nevertheless it echoes the World Health Organisation's principle that medical services have only a limited contribution to make towards health. The WHO declaration of Health For All 2000 outlined the importance of intersectoral cooperation:

"[Health For All] requires the coordinated action of all sectors concerned. The health authorities can deal only with a part of the problems to be solved and multisectoral cooperation is the only way of effectively ensuring the prerequisites for health, promoting health policies and reducing the risks in the physical, economic and social environment" (WHO, 1985).

As we saw in Chapter 2, although there has been a long term improvement in the overall health status of the population (measured by broad indicators such as life expectancy and infant mortality rates), the UK continues to suffer an avoidable burden of ill health and premature death. This is not evenly or randomly distributed across the population but is associated with factors such as socio-economic status and ethnic origin. A health strategy which addresses economic development is thus of vital importance.

Changes in the structure and management of health care have also prompted the move to a national strategy for health. The UK, although a signatory to the WHO "Health For All" targets, has until recently deemed health a matter for the NHS and refused to recommend a coordinated approach. However, the 1990 NHS and Community Care Act specifically charged the NHS with strategic responsibility for health promotion. The split between its "purchaser" and "provider" functions has highlighted the purchasing role as a major mechanism for achieving change and collaboration with other key agencies. Further information on the changes in the NHS and how these affect health promotion can be found at the end of this chapter.

Since the 1970s health authorities, local authorities and voluntary organizations have attempted to plan together services for "client groups" for whom health and local authorities were felt to have an interest such as the elderly or mentally ill. Since 1977 Joint Finance has been an allocation of funds specifically earmarked for projects jointly agreed between the participating organizations. However, the Intersectoral Collaboration and Health For All research project based at Leeds Metropolitan University has argued that the joint planning mechanisms of Joint Consultative Committees (JCC) and Joint Care Planning Teams (JCPT) take few decisions beyond their statutory responsibility to endorse proposals for Joint Finance expenditure, and there has been little strategic collaboration (Moran, 1990). However, with the shift towards "care in the community" of vulnerable groups, local and health authorities are required to publish joint community care plans and to purchase appropriate services.

Financial constraints on all organizations and the rising demand for services partly as a result of demographic change, has emphasized the need to assess existing patterns of resource use and the possibility of better collaboration.

☞ **There are at least three possible ways in which agencies may relate:**

1. Bureaucratic approach as in joint consultative committees and joint care planning teams.
2. Market mechanisms as in contracts between NHS and social services departments.
3. Association approach where co-operation arises out of common interests. In this case formal structures need to be differentiated from the wide range of formal and informal working links.

(Nocon, 1993)

The Healthy Cities Project began in the UK in 1986 following publication of the Health For All targets. More than 70 local authorities and 50 health authorities as well as voluntary organizations and academic institutions are involved (Faculty of Public Health Medicine of the Royal College of Physicians Health For All 2000 quarterly bulletin). The original aim of the Healthy Cities project was to provide opportunities for intersectoral collaboration in health promotion and develop models of good practice.

"Healthy Sheffield" was launched in 1987 as a joint initiative between the City Council, Community Health Council, Racial Equality Council, Family Health Services Authority (FHSA), Health Authority, Polytechnic and Voluntary Action Sheffield. Its aims were to improve the health of the people in Sheffield and reduce health inequalities. In order to achieve these aims "Healthy Sheffield" has sought to extend the partner agencies to all major organizations, and voluntary and community groups, many of whom had not identified their part in health promotion. It now includes both "old" and "new" universities, the Chamber of Commerce and the Trades Council. As its members expand, it has set up a support team whose role is to introduce the concepts and values of "Healthy Sheffield" to prospective partners helping them to embrace a holistic and social approach to health, and to clarify their own priorities in relation to health and the service they provide.

Another essential element for enabling change was the development of a range of demonstration projects and programmes to show what is possible in health promotion. Initially "Healthy Sheffield" found it difficult to progress beyond generalities when trying to apply HFA targets to Sheffield. An approach was then chosen which concentrates on the health needs of the main groups of people in the city and identifies priority targets for each group. This formed the structure for a major "Our City, Our Health" consultation exercise. This involved the training of over 200 facilitators to seek the views of their own colleagues and others. The consultation has been a political and educational process resulting in a document made accessible and readable for the community (Healthy Sheffield, 1990; Halliday and Adams, 1992).

Advantages of working together

Collaboration is a difficult challenge but, put simply, it creates "additionality". It brings together strengths and weaknesses, and makes something that exceeds the sum of the parts. Conventional wisdom favours group rather than individual decisions and phrases such as "two heads are better than one" reflect the view that better decisions are often made by people working together.

The advantages can be summarized as:

1. It brings together organizations and groups who would not normally see themselves as having a role in promoting health, and thus means that health is addressed holistically and not solely in a treatment-oriented setting.
2. It increases these organizations' knowledge and understanding of each other, helping to clarify roles and overcome rivalry.
3. Collaborative   service   planning   is   based   on   a   more

comprehensive picture of local needs. This will help to eliminate gaps.

4. It ensures accurate targeting of services based on wider consultation, and a pooling of knowledge and awareness of community needs.
5. Working in an alliance may lead to more effective use of resources by, for example, joint purchasing of services. It can also avoid administrative duplication by partners working together on service specifications.
6. It ensures the public are given the same, not conflicting, messages.
7. The root causes of ill health may be tackled, not just symptoms, and awareness can be raised of the determinants of ill health.

The experience of some collaborative projects, health strategy groups and "Healthy Cities" initiatives have not all been unqualified successes. Not surprisingly, these are not fully documented but there are some general barriers that can arise:

1. Lack of commitment at a senior level.
2. Differences in outlook.
3. Professional rivalry especially if there are differences in status.
4. Imbalance in the contributions to resourcing the alliance. Voluntary organizations, for example, are not able to contribute to the costs of intersectoral collaboration.
5. Exclusion of new partners.
6. Lack of appropriate skills.
7. Lack of shared, achievable goals.
8. Lack of understanding of different organizational cultures and the constraints of other organizations.
9. Different geographic boundaries, for example, between local authority and health authority.
10. Lack of real achievement.

> ☞ "Look After Your Heart Avon is a multi-agency heart disease prevention programme, cited as an example of good practice in 'Working Together for Better Health'. How has it survived? Probably because of personal commitment on the part of individual officers, who have hung on to the work despite all the changes. But this is a fragile basis for an alliance... What sticks in the throat is the syrupy coating on a once solid practice now being eaten away from the inside by the fragmentation and competition caused by market forces, lack of resources, and constant organisational change" (Ewles, 1993 p. 3)

A healthy alliance is a means not an end, and partnerships can fall apart, become "talking shops" or not make any decisions. These barriers can be overcome. The next section outlines the necessary features of a successful alliance.

Individuals and groups who work together will have perceptions of the other's role and may not understand the ways in which their organization works. This example illustrates the changing views of a health education coordinator from a local education authority and a youth worker from a drug project.

"We did have concerns about the reliability of the advice which might be given and the informal ways of working. We were worried what might be said that could be thought to be the Authority viewpoint. We were reassured by the response from young people who had not previously had the trust and confidence to express their needs." (Local education authority co-ordinator working with a voluntary drug project)

" At first we found the LEA very bureaucratic and hierarchical. Making the appropriate contacts was difficult. They seemed suspicious of our methods and our professionalism. Budget considerations and the corporate view seemed dominant. The success of the local drug education strategy has been because of individual effort and constant contact with those involved."
(Drug project worker)

Characteristics of successful joint working

Health promotion requires good team-work and coordination both with colleagues in your own department, but also with other disciplines and professions. In large organizations like health authorities or local authorities, it is especially important that there is good communication and coordination between departments because it is not always possible to have informal contacts or networking. Joint working does not happen easily and crossing professional lines is a difficult process perhaps involving rivalry, competing interests, different models of health or different ways of working. In addition, people may feel their own jobs to be threatened by joint working.

When people refer to a "good team", they usually mean a partnership in which the members work well together towards the same end and complement each other. An ideal team has certain essential characteristics:

■ A common task or purpose
■ Members are selected because they have specific expertise
■ Members know their own roles and those of other members
■ Members support each other in the task
■ Members complement each other in their skills and personalities
■ Members have a commitment to accomplishing the task
■ There is a leader who will coordinate and take responsibility
■ The team may have a base.

In addition, there are general skills of working with other people that contribute to a successful and "healthy" alliance. These skills include communication, participation in meetings, managing paperwork and time, and being and working in a group.

The Health of the Nation handbook (Department of Health, 1993) on healthy alliances identifies the following general factors as important:

Members must have sufficient time to devote to inter-agency activity otherwise it gets relegated by pressing and immediate professional concerns.

A co-ordinator may help to maintain commitment and to identify potential resources.

Members must have sufficient status and authority in their own organization to influence decisions otherwise collaboration becomes only a networking process.

There must be a shared vision and concept of health. Achieving this must be one of the first tasks of a healthy alliance. Most health authorities have a disease-related focus and most local authorities emphasize a behavioural approach. Some localities such as Sheffield explicitly state that their philosophy is that of a social model of health principally committed to reducing inequalities in health.

There must be shared goals and targets for promoting health. Some agencies may not be clear about their potential contribution or have their own objectives, interests and capacities. It is not uncommon for groups to spend years formulating operational targets which are relevant to local needs, realistic and compatible with the interests and business objectives of the individual partner agencies.

There must be support for collaboration and a mechanism for getting things done. Tangible results encourage people to keep working together.

It is important to demonstrate achievements. This may include monitoring the process of the alliance including levels of commitment and participation, and levels of activity. It may also measure outcomes and the achievement of original objectives.

? A Primary Health Care Team may consist of a GP, a practice manager, a receptionist, a practice nurse, a district nurse, a health visitor, a midwife, a social worker, a community psychiatric nurse, a dietitian, a chiropodist, a physiotherapist, a counsellor and an interpreter.

Consider some of the potential difficulties of these professions working together in a team:

1. There is no common task. All relate to the same registered population but activities range from episodes of illness in individuals, the care of the chronically ill and preventive activities for the whole population.
2. The membership will thus vary with the task. For example, a GP and district nurse may be the only members involved in the care of an elderly diabetic, whereas most of the above would be involved in the organization of a Well Woman Clinic.

(cont.)

3. There are boundary problems. Jobs frequently overlap and there are aspects of social and personal care that would seem to be part of all members' occupational remit.
4. There may be status problems. Within a Primary Health Care Team there are members who differ widely in the extent of their training, salary levels, degree of occupational autonomy and power.
5. Members have different employers which may result in different objectives. GPs are independent contractors who employ some team members, whereas others are employed by local or health authorities.

 Consider the following description of two posts in a health authority and in a local authority. Can you think of a similar example in your work of overlapping roles? How are boundary problems resolved?

From 1986–1993 the Department for Education contributed to the funding of local health and drug education coordinators whose role was to support and encourage programmes of health education in schools and colleges, particularly in relation to sexual health and substance use. Most health promotion units have a designated worker for schools whose role would be similar in its objectives. The different employers influence the nature of the work undertaken and its perspective. The local education authority health education co-ordinator is concerned with educational management and whole curriculum issues, whereas the health promotion officer has a specific brief for health programmes. There is also a considerable difference in salary scales though not necessarily any difference in experience or training undertaken. Because health education is frequently squeezed out of school education, health education specialists have to work to raise awareness and market their services.

The health education co-ordinator and the health promotion officer are employed in similar jobs. They may be healthy collaborators or healthy (or unhealthy) competitors.

Key stakeholders

As we have seen earlier in this chapter, local structures as well as personality and skills will determine which people and organizations contribute to a healthy alliance. The following will be key stakeholders in promoting health:

- Government departments
- Health authorities
- Health Education Authority
- Health promotion specialists
- Community nurses
- General practitioners
- Professions allied to medicine
- Local authorities
- Local education authorities

■ Community groups and voluntary organizations
■ Business sector and major employers
■ Mass media.

Figure 8.1 indicates the most important agencies of health promotion.

Any account of the current structure and organization of health promotion services is in danger of becoming out of date in the near future. However, a brief description is included to outline the opportunities for healthy alliances for each organization.

Government departments

The *Health of the Nation* emphasizes the potential contribution to health of many Government departments but mentions, in particular, the Home Office, the Department for Education, the Department of Health, the Department of the Environment, the Department of Social Security, the Department of Employment, the Department of Transport, and the Ministry of Agriculture, Fisheries and Food. Inter-departmental committees exist for HIV/AIDS prevention and drug misuse, but otherwise co-operation seems fragmented. Arguably it is economic policy which has the biggest single influence on the nation's health by affecting levels of employment, by adopting taxation policies which are regressive and affect everyone (such as increases in VAT rather than income tax), and by a reliance on the £12 billion raised in alcohol and tobacco revenue each year.

Health authorities

There are currently 14 regional health authorities in England and Wales whose role is to implement policy and oversee the establishment of contracts which give people access to health services. They allocate resources and monitor the performance of district health authorities and family health service authorities. The regional health authorities are, in turn, responsible to the NHS Executive. From 1994 these will be reduced to 8 NHS Management Executive Regional Offices with a lesser role, mainly confined to staffing and the supervision of contracts.

The NHS and Community Care Act 1990 divided health authorities into "purchasers" and "providers". The purchasing authority has responsibility for determining health needs and commissioning services from provider units.

District health authorities (DHAs) are the main purchasers of health care. DHAs have to assess the health needs of their population and then agree service contracts with provider units,

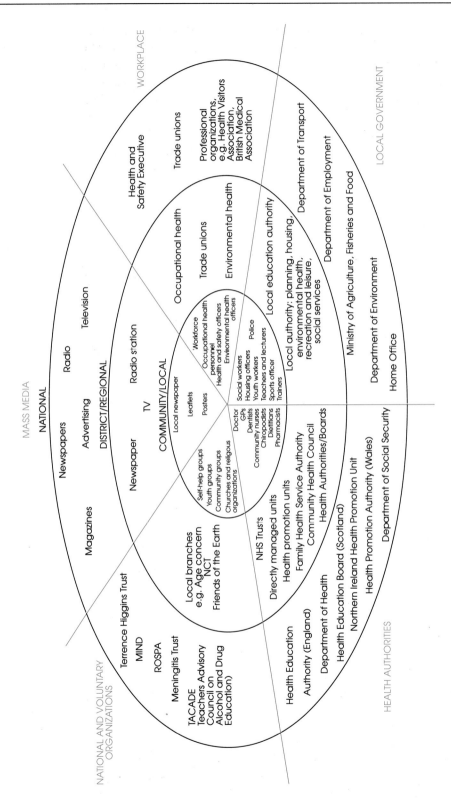

Figure 8.1 Agencies of health promotion

which may be hospitals or community services within the DHA, self-governing hospitals, or other health authorities (see Table 8.1). The DHA can purchase services outside the health service and is increasingly working with other agencies to deliver essential services. They are also having to become more responsive to their "clients" – identifying and setting out the views of service users, and specifying quality standards in their contracts with hospitals and other providers of care. Chapter 11 looks at the ways in which DHAs are having to use a wide range of research techniques and "intelligence gathering" in order to build a picture of needs in their community.

Putting health into contracts and service specifications may include:

- A requirement of all provider units to provide a certain standard of health education and promotion in patient care such as ensuring a smoke-free environment.
- A requirement to promote the health of NHS employees such as the provision of healthy catering.
- Specifications that define the co-ordinating and support role of a provider, usually the health promotion unit.
- A requirement for providers to use health needs assessment, to encourage the active participation of users and other members of the community in the planning of services, and to observe equal opportunities (Killoran, 1992).

Table 8.1 The health care market.

Purchasers	
Regional health authorities	Assess the need for health care
District health authorities	Develop service specifications
Family health service authorities	Establish contracts
GP budget holders	Monitor the health of the population
Providers	
Directly managed units	Provide services under contract with their
NHS trusts	own or other districts
Private sector	Negotiate the price of services
Voluntary sector	Generate income
Local authorities	

The Director of Public Health is a relatively new role established in 1988 following the publication of the Acheson report on public health in England (Acheson, 1988). The role is far broader than the previous District Medical Officer or before that, the Medical Officers of Health who were employed by the local authority. The Director of Public Health is charged with assessing overall health needs, collaborating with other agencies in the promotion of health and prevention of disease, and producing an annual report on the state of public health locally.

Community nurses

Health promotion is a priority in the role of community nurses, and is written into the job specification of health visitors and school nurses (Health Visitors Association, 1987). Their work is to promote the health of their clients as well as specific care and monitoring tasks. Because community nurses visit people in their own homes, they are able to build a strong relationship with their clients over a period of time. This enables them to carry out much one-to-one education, and counselling and opportunistic health education. Some nurses are also involved with supporting community and voluntary groups working in health-related areas.

Community nurses are part of the Primary Health Care Team and should work closely with other community nurses, GPs and social workers. The planning of health promotion may not always be co-ordinated or prioritized, however, as each health care worker concentrates on their case load. The potential for health promotion is discussed further in the section on Primary Health Care in Chapter 13.

Health visitors

Health visitors have a duty to visit all mothers and new infants. Some may have smaller case loads and have additional responsibility for older people. Health visitors may run antenatal classes and postnatal support groups in addition to carrying out health checks for the under-fives and providing support and advice for parents.

District nurses

District nurses visit people with chronic sickness or disability at home. Much of their work is with older people, and they carry out opportunistic health education as well as liaising between people living in the community, and other relevant health and welfare workers.

Community psychiatric nurses

Community psychiatric nurses visit people who are mentally ill and ensure that they are coping. They may be involved with self-help groups or mental health education in addition to having a client caseload.

Community midwives

Community midwives visit all new mothers in their area, and provide support and education as well as monitoring the health of mothers and babies.

?

Kensington, Chelsea, Westminster and Brent (previously Parkside) has a health promotion forum consisting of: health visitors working on a locality basis; a health visitor for ethnic minority groups, a health visitor for homeless families, a parentcraft co-ordinator, a health promotion officer; a community pharmacist; and a community dietitian. The aim of the forum is to encourage partnerships with community groups and reorientate their service to meet the needs of the community.

Consider the range of community groups that each member could access. It includes:

- An antenatal group for the homeless community
- A child-minder's group
- A women's refuge
- A weight group
- A pensioner's group
- NSPCC
- Moroccan women's group; an Arab women's group; a Bengali women's group
- Parentcraft groups
- Sickle cell group
- Family service unit drop-in
- Schools.

Health promotion units

Health promotion units are part of the district health authority and are usually accountable to the Director of Public Health. They vary widely in size from a handful to 50 staff, and will consist of health promotion specialists and several support and clerical staff. They have the lead role in initiating, coordinating, and supporting health education and health promotion activity. Health promotion units may have purchasing or providing functions, or a dual role.

Purchaser activities include:

- Assessing local health needs
- Contributing to the operational and strategic plans of the DHA
- Reviewing contracts to ensure they seek to *promote* health
- Co-ordinating the plans and services of different agencies.

Provider activities include:

- Managing health education/health promotion programmes on specific issues such as HIV/AIDS, smoking or coronary heart disease.

■ Providing advice and consultancy to the public and policy makers.

■ Providing training, support, and advice to all health promotion specialists and agencies who provide health promotion.

Family health service authority

The FHSA replaced the previous Family Practitioner Committee. The FHSA plans the provision of services and manages the contracts of GPs, dentists, pharmacists and opticians, and monitors the provision of health promotion. FHSAs provide training and support for health promotion in primary health care through, for example, funding primary health care facilitators.

Community health councils

Community health councils (CHCs) were set up under the 1974 NHS reorganization to give a stronger voice to the views of the community on health services. CHCs have representatives from voluntary groups, local authorities and community groups. They act as a lobby group and will also participate in the NHS planning process. Their future is uncertain.

General practice

General practice has traditionally been a private and personal consultation between doctor and patient. Health promotion consisted of opportunistic advice or information. GPs are essentially independent practitioners administered by the FHSA. The Government White Paper *Promoting Better Health* (DHSS, 1987), however, emphasized the role of GPs in prevention and the monitoring of chronic illness. Revised contracts now provide additional payments to GPs to carry out preventive work. Details of the new GP contracts are included in the section on Primary Health Care in Chapter 13.

Dentists

There is an increasing emphasis on prevention in dentistry particularly with children. Dentists receive a capitation fee per child and so have an interest in keeping that child's teeth healthy and free from treatment. Many practices employ a hygienist who will give advice on dental health. Health authorities also have a community dental service which may offer dental health promotion to schools and residential homes.

Professions allied to medicine

Many other professions allied to medicine such as chiropodists and dietitians have a part to play in health promotion, and particularly patient education. The expanded role of the community pharmacist is used here as an example.

Pharmacists

There are nearly 12 000 community pharmacists in the UK which thus provide an ideal and easily accessible location for the provision of opportunistic health promotion advice. Pharmacists have always offered education about medication and patient counselling when prescription medicines are required. The priority accorded to health promotion is now much higher. Pharmacists may offer education about specific health issues when products are purchased. For example, pharmacists are active in raising awareness about skin cancer. There are also opportunities for opportunistic health advice. The client purchasing a laxative may be invited to discuss their diet and sources of fibre.

There have been several pharmacy-based campaigns. The DUMP scheme encourages the public to return unwanted medicines. The "Health Care in the High Street" is a joint initiative by the Health Education Authority, the Family Planning Association, the National Pharmaceutical Association and the Royal Pharmaceutical Society of Great Britain. It aims to develop the community pharmacy as an information centre for general health advice.

Pharmacists have not necessarily been trained in health promotion or communication skills, nor are they paid for health promotion work. The pharmacist is not generally seen by the public as a source of health advice apart from on medication (MarPlan, 1982). However, *Promoting Better Health* (DHSS, 1987) and a Nuffield Report on the future of pharmacists (Nuffield Foundation, 1986) both suggest an extension of their role and closer links with other professionals, particularly in the primary health care team so that pharmacists work with their clients' health not their illness, and with the person not their condition.

 This is an example of collaboration on an exercise project "Prescription for Exercise" between health promotion, leisure services, FHSA and a GP practice.

Clients at risk of coronary heart disease, at a check-up may be offered, if appropriate, a prescription for exercise. This gives information on types of recommended activities and a list of leisure centres. The "prescription" can be handed in at a centre and the client can take part in activities at reduced cost. The referring GP will monitor the patient at intervals of 1 and 3 months.

Health Education Authority

The HEA is part of the NHS and is designated a "special" health authority with the task of leading and supporting health education in England. In Scotland, the Health Education Board carries out this function. In Wales, it is the Health Promotion Authority and in Northern Ireland it is the Northern Ireland Health Promotion Unit.

☞ **The role of the HEA is:**

■ To give information and advice about health directly to the public
■ To support other health organizations, health professionals and other people who give health education to the public (usually by training or the provision of resources)
■ To advise Government on matters related to health.

By contrast, in Wales there is a Health Promotion Authority. This followed the establishment in 1985 of Heartbeat Wales, a project to test the feasibility of a major health promotion exercise in the field of cardiovascular disease prevention on a regional basis along the lines of the North Karelia project (WHO, 1981) and the Stanford Health Project in the USA. Heartbeat Wales has sought to bring about structural changes, for example, restrictions on smoking in public places, better food labelling, including the provision of healthy foods in shops and canteens. It has worked closely with the mass media, sometimes buying "air time" or space, but more usually highlighting research data or specific achievements.

The contrasting aims and priority accorded to health promotion is highlighted by the difference in budget. In England, the HEA spent 0.5p per head of population in 1989. In Wales, the Health Promotion Authority spent 10p per head (National Audit Office, 1989).

Local authorities

Local authorities include county, district, borough and metropolitan authorities which provide a range of services for local communities. Local authority officers are accountable to elected councillors who represent the local community.

Some authorities are major providers of housing. Most are major employers. Individual departments also have key roles in the promotion of health: social services, recreation and leisure, planning, housing and environmental health (HEA, 1991). The responsibility local authorities have for transport provides the opportunity for initiatives on accident prevention and environmental schemes, such as park and ride or bike lanes.

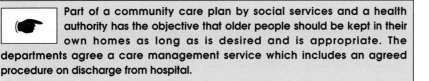

The role of environmental health is particularly wide ranging, encompassing statutory powers relating to food hygiene and pollution (both of noise and air) to specialist work on safety in the workplace and places of entertainment. Because the environmental health officer has wide-ranging statutory powers, their work in health promotion is mainly advice on legislation and enabling people to fulfil those regulations. Their work may thus involve offering training courses or one-to-one advice in establishments.

City of London and Westminster Home Safety Council is an example of the way groups can work together. Partners include the local authority, the Metropolitan Police, London Fire Brigade, the utility companies and many businesses. The group has:

- Put smoke alarms in local authority homes for older people
- Introduced grants for home safety equipment
- Developed a training programme on home safety for health visitors, social workers, child-minders, playgroup leaders and foster carers.

The emphasis on the public sector offering contracts for its services rather than necessarily being providers themselves has given it wide opportunities to promote positive health in its service specifications.

Social services

The shift towards care in the community under the 1990 NHS and Community Care Act has increased the role of social services in promoting the health of older people, people with mental health problems, those with learning difficulties and people with a disability. The new legislation requires social service departments to work with health authorities to provide individualized care programmes for people in need in these groups, and also people with AIDS or drug or alcohol problems.

Part of a community care plan by social services and a health authority has the objective that older people should be kept in their own homes as long as is desired and is appropriate. The departments agree a care management service which includes an agreed procedure on discharge from hospital.

Social service departments already have a statutory responsibility for child protection and, under the Children Act 1989, a responsibility to provide a health-promoting environment for young people in its care. Social service departments may also be taking a major role in sexual health promotion, and drug and alcohol education and prevention.

Local education authorities

The LEA has responsibility for health education in schools, colleges and youth clubs. Over 6 million young people between the ages of five and 19 are in education. Over 3 million teenagers attend a youth club. Education is therefore a key setting for health education and promotion. There have been many recent changes in the management of education which have devolved budgets directly to schools and given governors greater powers. Governors are responsible under the 1986 Education (No.2) Act for the provision of sexual health education. The introduction of the National Curriculum in schools in 1989 has meant that health education is often squeezed out of an overcrowded timetable. This process has been exacerbated by the disbanding of the LEA specialist advisors for health education. On the other hand, there is far greater recognition of the importance of health education and many schools have a designated teacher co-ordinator. The opportunities for health promotion in schools is discussed more fully in Chapter 13.

A similar problem occurs in colleges where the huge increase in student numbers and vocational courses in recent years has meant a squeeze on pastoral time and non-vocational studies. The only health education for this age group is often advice or counselling sought by the student from a counselling service.

Personal and social education has always been central to the work of the youth service. Increasingly educational activity is offered alongside the traditional games and sports. These moves are encouraged by the debate over a proposed curriculum for youth work which would specify work on, for example, sexuality and substance use.

Voluntary sector

There are numerous voluntary agencies ranging from large organizations with paid staff and budgets to small groups run by volunteers. Many have an interest in health ranging from MIND (the National Association for Mental Health) or Age Concern to agencies concerned with particular conditions, such as the Alzheimer's Society, to established projects staffed by paid workers in fields such as substance use, for example, Turning Point.

Voluntary organizations are involved in statutory structures such as Joint Consultative Committees and Community Health Councils, and in planning and consultation exercises, such as the Community Care Plan of the health authority and local authority.

Voluntary organizations are important in providing specialized information, being close to the community and harder to reach groups. They can reflect people's experience of a service and give an indicator of other needs acting as a catalyst for change.

The development of the purchaser/provider role in the NHS and towards a mixture of health and social care services will necessitate good relations between statutory and voluntary sectors. However, the precarious funding of many voluntary organizations which need to be engaged in a constant search for grants can make long-term planning difficult and lead to low morale. Many organizations now require that any collaborative exercise is purchased by the relevant statutory authority.

 The Brent Sickle Cell and Thalassaemia Centre provides an example of mutual respect and effective collaboration between statutory and voluntary sectors.

This service was set up in 1980 for those affected by sickle cell disorders. It includes the screening of babies and adults, genetic and general counselling, health promotion advice on nutrition and welfare issues. The centre is funded by the regional health authority and is part of health service provision. However, it is based in a small, easily accessible hospital and operates an open-door policy with no appointments. It is so sensitive to the needs of the local community and works so closely with the volunteer parents support group that it is often seen as a black voluntary organization. Its workers regard this as an achievement and a breaking down of barriers.

The centre relies on networking between volunteers, patients and health professionals and overlapping roles. Thus counselling is carried out by nurses, health visitors and volunteers. The local support group meets in the centre and uses its facilities.

Source: Fieldgrass, 1992.

Workplace

In the workplace trade unions may have an active role in health promotion. However, membership of unions has declined dramatically in the last decade. Traditionally, unions have protected rather than promoted their members' health, and have been more concerned with safety factors and environmental hazards than the general work environment. Similarly, but for different reasons, employers and managers have been concerned with safety conditions and the efficient working of staff rather than promoting their health. The potential and limitations are discussed further in the section on workplace health promotion in Chapter 13.

Large employers will have an occupational health scheme which may provide health checks, health promotion advice as well as first aid. Health and safety officers are responsible for ensuring that workplaces conform to safety legislation.

Mass media

Health promotion messages are presented in a variety of media including print or visual media produced by health promoters themselves, newspaper features or news, magazine advice columns, or health pages, radio phone-ins, and fictional television programmes. As Chapter 13 outlines, the role of health promoters in using the media and making it part of a "healthy alliance" is still limited. This is despite the traditional use of advertising-type campaigns to present simple behavioural messages.

> **?** **Skin cancer (malignant melanoma) is associated with exposure to ultraviolet radiation. Deaths from skin cancer account for 1% of all cancer deaths and 4% of all cancer deaths in the 0–44 age group.**
>
> Which of the above organizations and agencies would you expect to involve in a prevention strategy?

Conclusion

Intersectoral collaboration is one of the key principles outlined by the WHO if Health For All is to be achieved. It is not sufficient alone, however, to reduce inequalities or reorientate health services, or catalyse and persuade communities to actively participate in their own health decisions. Chapter 9 goes on to look at community development approaches to health promotion and the consultation, training, support and resources that are necessary if there is to be a local health-oriented programme.

Questions for further discussion

What are the prospects and problems of working with others to promote health in your work?

Summary

This chapter has explored different examples of healthy alliances and ways in which health promotion specialists can work together. It discussed the conditions that are necessary for effective collaboration concluding that coordination and a greater understanding of other workers' roles would greatly enhance intersectoral collaboration. It then outlined the role and potential of the main agencies that promote health.

Further reading

Davies J, Dooris M, Russell J and Petersson G (1993) *Healthy Alliances: A Study of Inter-agency Collaboration in Health Promotion*, London, South West Thames Regional Health Authority.

Despite the emphasis on collaboration in health promotion, there is little written material. This study of the process of inter-agency collaboration on accident prevention, coronary heart disease prevention and a young people's programme is thoroughly researched and makes interesting reading.

Department of Health (1993) *Working Together for Better Health*, London, HMSO

A handbook produced as part of the Health of the Nation strategy. It summarizes the reasons for working together, how to organize a healthy alliance, whom to involve and provides many case studies which set out the benefits for those involved.

English National Board for Nursing (ENB) (1989) *Health Promotion in Primary Health Care*, Learning Materials Design, ENB.

An open learning package for practice nurses which is well designed and stimulating.

Fieldgrass J (1992) *Partnerships in Health Promotion*, London, HEA.

A summary of existing partnerships between the NHS and voluntary organizations.

Health Education Authority (1991) *Promoting Health –*

Local Authorities in Action London, HEA.

This report also includes a summary of the role of statutory agencies and their contribution to health promotion.

Rolls L (1992) *Team Development: a Manual of Facilitation for Health Educators and Health Promoters*, London, HEA.

A practical and useful guide for building teams.

Seedhouse D and Cribb A (1989) *Changing Ideas in Health Care*, Chichester, Wiley.

A collection of articles on health initiatives which emphasize holism and arise from a wide range of disciplines. The book shows how practice is being reorientated.

References

Acheson D (1988) *Public Health in England*, Report of the Committee of Inquiry into the Future Development of the Public Health Function, London, HMSO.

Department of Health (1992) *The Health of the Nation*, London, HMSO.

Department of Health (1993) *Working Together for Better Health*, London, HMSO.

DHSS (1987) *Promoting Better Health*, London, HMSO.

Ewles L (1993) *Hope Against Hope. Health Service Journal*, 26 August, 30–31.

Halliday M and Adams L (1992) "Healthy Sheffield: the consultation experiment", *Health Education Journal*, **51**, 1.

Health Education Authority (1991) Promoting Health – Local Authorities in Action, London, HEA.

Healthy Sheffield (1990) *Health Promotion Strategic Plan 1990–1993*.

Health Visitors Association (HVA) (1987) *Health Visiting and School Nursing Reviewed*, London, HVA.

Killoran A (1992) *Putting Health into Contracts*, London, HEA.

MarPlan (1982) *Survey of Public Attitudes and Knowledge Carried Out on Behalf of the National Pharmaceutical Association*, London, NPA.

Moran G (1990) *Local Collaboration in Health Promotion*, Paper for the Intersectoral Collaboration and Health For All Project, Leeds Polytechnic.

National Audit Office (1989) *NHS: Coronary Heart Disease*, London, HMSO.

Nocon A (1993) Made in Heaven? *Health Service Journal*, 2 December 24–26.

Nuffield Foundation (1986) *Pharmacy: The Report of a Committee of Inquiry Appointed by the Nuffield Foundation*, London, Nuffield.

World Health Organisation (1981) *Community Control of Cardiovascular Diseases: the North Karelia Project*, Copenhagen, WHO.

World Health Organisation (1985) *Targets for Health for All*, Copenhagen, WHO Regional Office for Europe.

9 Working with communities and community development

Overview

We have seen in previous chapters how working with communities to increase their participation in decisions affecting health is an essential aspect of health promotion. There are many terms used to describe ways of working with communities. Community involvement, community participation, community action and community development are all commonly applied to health promotion, and are often used interchangeably. This chapter begins by defining what is meant by a community and goes on to explore different ways in which health promoters can work with communities. Some of the dilemmas that confront the health promoter who wants to work in this way are discussed and illustrated using examples of community development projects.

Key points
- Defining community development
- Community development in health promotion
- Community development as a radical approach
- Dilemmas for practice

What is the community?

- Which communities do you belong to?
- Are these the same communities which your parents belonged to?
- What are the key characteristics of these communities?

The concept of community is frequently used in discussions about health and health care. In general, the context of the community is taken to be desirable; thus we have care in the community, community policing, and community education, all of which are seen as preferable to alternative (non-community) practice. In contrast to the state or the bureaucratic organization, services provided by and in the community are viewed as being more appropriate and sensitive. But what is the community which is referred to in these ways?

There are different ways of defining the community, but the most commonly cited factors are geography, culture and social stratification. These factors are viewed as being linked to the subjective feeling of belonging or identity which characterizes the concept of "community". Other characteristics of communities are social networks or systems of contact, and the existence of potential resources such as people's skills or knowledge.

Geography

A community may be defined on a geographical or neighbourhood basis. A well-known example is the East End of London, but this use of community is not restricted to working class or urban areas. It is this notion of community which gives rise to "patch" based work, where people such as social workers, police officers or health visitors are assigned a geographically bounded area. The assumption is that people living in the same area have the same concerns, owing to their geographical proximity.

Culture

Community may be defined in cultural terms, as in "the Chinese community" or "the Jewish community". Here the assumption is that common cultural traditions may transcend geographical or other barriers, and unite otherwise scattered and disparate groups of people. There is an expectation that members of a cultural community will assist each other and share resources. The most commonly cited elements of a common cultural heritage are ethnic origin, language, religion and customs.

Social stratification

A community may be based on interests held to be common, which are usually the product of social stratification. Thus we have "the working class community" and "the gay community". This definition implies that members of a community share networks of support, knowledge and resources which may transcend other boundaries even national ones.

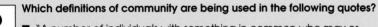

? **Which definitions of community are being used in the following quotes?**

- "A number of individuals with something in common who may or may not acknowledge that connection" (HEA, 1987)
- "A locality which comprises networks of formal and informal relationships, which have a capacity to mobilise individual and collective responses to common adversity" (Barclay Report, 1982)
- "People with a basis of common interest and network of personal interaction, grouped either on the basis of locality or on a specific shared concern or both" (Smithies and Adams 1990, p. 9).

Most definitions of community tend to suggest it is an homogeneous entity. However, it is obvious that any geographical community will include people whose primary identity is based on different factors, e.g. class, race, gender or sexual orientation. And people who feel united by a shared interest, e.g. pensioners, or the unemployed, will also be members of other communities, geographical and otherwise. People may belong to several different communities, some of which may have more salience for the individual than others. In practice, people may find their allegiance to different communities shifting at different points in their life span.

Guidelines for adoption state that couples should provide positive role models and reflect the ethnic origins of the child. A mixed race couple seeking to adopt an Asian baby were turned down when the Asian woman reported no experience of racism or discrimination.

■ What definition of identity, and hence community, is being used?
■ Whose definition is being used?

This example demonstrates how professionally imposed notions of cultural community may be experienced by clients as coercive rather than enabling.

The meaning and significance of community varies enormously. How one defines community is important because it influences how community representatives may be identified and communicated with.

Definition of terms

Community development

Following Smithies and Adams (1990), we shall use the term community development to refer to "activity which arises from, and is controlled by, communities in order to empower a continually widening circle of participants" (Smithies and Adams, 1990, p.10).

Community participation

The involvement of people in the community in the formal processes of policy making and implementation. Participation can vary from high to low levels of involvement.

Outreach

Outreach is the extension of a professional service into the community in order to make it more accessible. The location may be in the community, but there is no challenge to professional norms or claim to expertise. Outreach work is determined by professional priorities and the focus is on obtaining certain outcomes defined by professionals. An example of outreach is a mobile bus offering cervical cancer screening to women at their place of work. This may increase uptake of services by making them more accessible, but the type of service provision is predetermined and is not open for negotiation.

Community health projects

Projects organized to meet people's health needs in the community. Projects may be independent, for example, self-help or voluntary projects, or located within the statutory services.

The history of community development

Community development has a long history dating back to the 19th century when it was used as a means of controlling Britain's colonies. In Britain community associations were linked to new housing areas built following the First World War. Rifkin (1990) argues that community participation in health care came to the forefront in developing countries after the Second World War. The newly independent ex-colonies became disillusioned with the Western medical system. The Western focus on a costly and technologically sophisticated infrastructure devoted to cure was seen as inappropriate and ineffective for their health needs. There was also a realization that public health policy is not a discrete area but forms an integral part of general social policy.

During the 1960s, poverty was rediscovered in the industrialized world. This led to programmes designed to alleviate the effects of poverty, such as Project Headstart (a pre-school education programme for deprived children) in the USA and the community development projects in Britain. In 1969 the Home Office funded 12 community development projects to work in areas of multiple deprivation. These areas were selected by professionals and the project was based on a number of assumptions. These were:

■ That deprived people were the cause of the problem
■ that self-help, organization and information could solve the problem
■ that action-research could lead to changes in policy
■ and that all parties involved would agree about priorities, values, and strategies.

The project had its funding withdrawn when it was found that the assumption of consensus was being disrupted. Community development workers were developing a conflict model of action, advocating a structural critique and radical solutions to problems. In a nutshell, they were being "too political" and were threatening to disrupt the consensus view (Green and Chapman, 1991).

Another important influence was Freire's theories about education for liberation. For Freire, learning grows out of reflection and leads to action. The starting point is the process of "cultural synthesis" (Freire, 1972), which is when activists and the people meet as equals, and develop a dialogue based on trust. This leads to critical consciousness raising which itself involves different stages:

- Reflection on aspects of reality
- Search and collective identification of the root causes of that reality
- An examination of their implications
- Development of a plan of action to change reality.

Critical consciousness is therefore an agent of revolutionary change. So from this viewpoint, community development is allied to revolution, and is a highly politicized and political activity.

The women's movement, and Black and ethnic minority groups have also been identified as factors underpinning community development in health (Jones, 1991). Health has been a central concern of the Women's Movement, which developed during the 1960s and 1970s. The Women's Health Movement emphasized the need to reclaim knowledge, especially knowledge about our bodies. Shared personal experience leads to a new understanding of health issues. Such knowledge results from women meeting together in supportive groups characterized by non-hierarchical structures. Black and ethnic minority groups have also addressed health issues, particularly the effect of racism within the health services.

Experiential learning, where learning results from reflecting on one's own experience, is a central strategy in community development. Such learning is most effective when it is shared with others, for example, through group discussion of health needs and priorities. It has a practical focus and leads to action to change reality.

Community development in health promotion

Community development has been defined as:

> "a process by which a community identifies its needs or objectives, orders (or ranks) these needs or objectives, develops the confidence and will to work at these needs or objectives, finds the resources (internal and/or external) to deal with these needs or objectives, takes action in respect to them, and in so doing extends and develops co-operative and collaborative attitudes and practices in the community" (Ross, 1955).

Community development for health is:

> "a process by which a community defines its own health needs, considers how those needs can be met and decides collectively on priorities for action" (CHIRU/LCHR, 1987).

Community development is a recurring theme in health promotion.

"The people have a right and a duty to participate individually and collectively in the planning and implementation of their health care" (WHO, 1978).

"Health for all will be achieved by people themselves. A well informed, well motivated and actively *participating community* is a key element for the attainment of the common goal" (WHO, 1985, p.5, original emphasis).

"Health promotion works through concrete and effective community action in setting priorities, making decisions, planning strategies and implementing them to achieve better health. At the heart of this process is the empowerment of communities, their ownership and control of their own endeavors and destinies" (WHO, 1986).

More recently, it has been claimed that empowering the community is the essence of health promotion (Green and Raeburn, 1990) and that community development is the central defining strategy for health promotion. Community development marks a shift away from the authoritarian medical model of health towards a collaborative social model of positive health.

Terms like community development and empowerment began to be commonplace in health promotion in the 1980s. The HEA set up a community and professional development division in 1988, but this was disbanded in 1990 after the resignation of its director. Community development and participation is now included as an arm of HEA priority programmes such as 'Look After Your Heart' (HEA, 1991). The community as such does not, however, figure as a key setting in *The Health of the Nation* (Department of Health, 1992). Instead, cities, schools, hospitals, workplaces, homes and environments are listed as key settings which "offer between them the potential to involve most people in the country" (Department of Health, 1992, p.26). But some people may miss out on interventions located in these settings. Where, for example, would the unemployed be targeted? Or travellers? These settings address people in certain ascribed roles located in certain social organizations. Thus we can reach young people in schools, workers in the workplace, and patients in hospitals. They do not address the whole person whose life straddles different settings and communities.

The community development approach is challenging. It offers the prospect of change for health but there are many practical difficulties to overcome.

Table 9.1 Advantages and disadvantages of the community development approach.

Advantages	Disadvantages
Starts with people's concerns, so it is more likely to gain support	Time consuming
Focuses on root causes of ill health, not symptoms	Results are often not tangible or quantifiable
Creates awareness of the social causes of ill health	Evaluation is difficult
The process of involvement is enabling and leads to greater confidence	Without evaluation, gaining funding is difficult
The process includes acquiring skills which are transferable, for example, communication skills, lobbying skills	The health promoter may find his or her role contradictory. To whom are they ultimately accountable – employer or community?
If health promoter and people meet as equals, it extends principle of democratic accountability	Work is usually with small groups of people

User led

In contrast to professionally determined priorities, community development starts with priorities identified by communities. This means starting out with people's concepts of health which are typically more broadly based than those of health workers. Coulter (1987) found that working-class people identified social, economic and environmental factors, such as unemployment, pollution, housing and income, as the most important influences on their health. (This is discussed in greater detail in Chapter 1.) Health is viewed holistically. Watt and Rodmell (1988) argue that this is the defining characteristic of community development and that the challenge this poses to medical dominance is its most important function. In particular, the social aspects of health are recognized as being of crucial importance:

> "Social networks have functions that are relevant to health... These health-relevant functions can be summarized in the concepts social support, social action, network promotion and empowerment" (Trojan *et al.*, 1991, p.449).

Focus on process

The process of enabling communities to promote health is viewed as a positive activity in its own right. Community development entails greater participation, and this process will itself enhance self-confidence, self-esteem and feelings of being in control, which are themselves health-promoting factors. Whether this activity is directed towards a specific health issue such as coronary heart disease, or more general issues, such as transport or housing, is not crucial, for the skills which are gained are transferable to different contexts.

■ How important do you think community development is as a health promotion strategy?
■ How does it compare with other approaches such as the medical preventive, individual empowerment, educational, behaviour change or social change approaches?

Activity with disadvantaged groups

The third characteristic is that community development acknowledges health inequalities and prioritizes activity with disadvantaged groups. Instead of focusing on individual lifestyles, community development focuses on the social determinants of ill health. This is seen as a more satisfactory means of promoting health, because it tackles the roots of the problem and avoids blaming the victim:

> ". . . while individuals come and go from deprived areas, the underlying social conditions which are largely responsible for their excessive amount of ill health remain the same" [Research Unit in Health Behaviour Change, 1989, p.126].

It is only by focusing on the underlying social conditions which reproduce ill health that the vicious cycle of illness and premature death can be broken. This has long been recognized by people living in deprived environments (Mitchell, 1984; Roberts, 1990). Community development is a professional strategy which sanctions this focus on structural inequalities.

These characteristics of community development have ensured its inclusion in the repertoire of health-promotion strategies.

Community development has been prioritized on the grounds of ethics and effectiveness. Community development is seen as embodying ethical principles such as autonomy and equality. It provides a means of avoiding "victim-blaming", and of tackling the root causes of ill health, not its symptoms. It is also viewed as a more effective means of health promotion:

> "not only is participation in decisions affecting health a right, but also a common sense approach, as the more that people feel involved in identifying their own health needs and shaping solutions, the more likely that the resulting action will be successful" (Sheffield Health for All, undated, cited in Roberts, 1992).

Types of activities involved in community development

A large number of different activities may be included in the term community development. Smithies and Adams (1990) propose five different categories of community action in health. These are:

- Formal participation in decision-making mechanisms
- Community action
- Facilitating processes which enable the community
- Professional and community interface
- Strategic support.

Formal participation

Formal participation may be thought of as a spectrum which includes many different activities. At the low or weak end, it may mean consultation to "rubber stamp" plans already drawn up by official agencies. At the high or strong end of the spectrum, it may mean control over the setting of priorities and implementation of programmes.

Community action

Community action is any activity undertaken by a community in order to effect change. This includes lobbying authorities to provide services, and the provision of voluntary or self-help services to address needs.

Trojan *et al.* (1991) conducted a survey of about 1700 community organizations in Hamburg. The findings of the survey were that between 75% and 85% of all health-related community organizations were actively engaged in providing social support, undertaking social action for better health, supporting networks within communities, and seeking to empower people. These activities are all important to health promotion. They conclude that "To a great extent, therefore, promoting health means strengthening community organizations" (Trojan *et al.*, 1991, p. 456).

Facilitating processes

Facilitating processes are those activities which are designed to increase and enhance people's skills in working for change. This may include providing appropriate training, and developing and supporting viable networks within communities.

Professional and community interface

Professional and community interface needs to be open and flexible if community development is to achieve real change. This can be achieved by a reorientation of professionals and official agencies so that community concerns are seen as legitimate. Organizational culture tends to be inward-looking, and this needs to be changed so that community views are actively sought and valued as part of the planning and provision of services.

Strategic support

Strategic support refers to organizational policies and initiatives which endorse community development and enable it to take place. Strategic support may function at different levels, neighbourhood, city, region or nationwide.

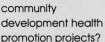

■ What positive outcomes have been attributed to community development health promotion projects?
■ Are these outcomes unique to community development?

The work of the Bristol Inner City Health Project during 1986–1990 included the following:

■ Secured agreement from the health authority to the setting up of a management group to increase community representation in the running of the project
■ Helped to set up an Asian self-help group for families with children with special needs
■ Appointed a welfare rights worker to provide advice about benefit entitlement in a health centre
■ Ran an anti-racist training course at a health centre for health care workers
■ Funded and supported a pilot project, "Health Links", under the umbrella of an existing organization, "Maternity Links". "Maternity Links" provides interpreting and advocacy services for non-English-speaking women around childbirth. "Health Links" extended this scheme to cover other patients' interpreting and advocacy needs
■ Supported the development of a health authority sickle cell policy
■ Evaluated the progress of all activities

Source: Beattie, 1991.

Community development: revolution or reform?

Community development has been applauded by people aligned on both the right and the left of the political spectrum.

For someone on the right, community development is associated with the idea of self-help, which in turn is linked to central values such as the exercise of free choice and self-determination. Community development may also be valued as a means of reducing state expenditure on services.

For someone on the left, community development is seen as a means of redressing the power imbalance by enabling communities to take more power and control over their environment and lives (RUHBC, 1989; Smithies and Adams, 1990). Community development is a means of identifying and acting on structural causes of inequality such as class, race and gender. It is also a means of increasing participation in formal decision-making processes and therefore of extending in practice the principle of democratic accountability. These principles are associated with the political values of the left, and in general, community development is associated with the values and practice of the political left.

■ Why might someone on the political left support community development?
■ Why might someone on the political right do the same?

However, it has been argued that community development maintains and reproduces the power differentials which currently exist. The literature concerning community development is unanimous in stating that the first priority is to determine community needs. Only when needs have been defined can ways of meeting these needs be devised. However, Armstrong (1982, p. 26, original emphasis) points out that ". . . 'needs' are *created* in the attempt to objectify a subjective desire or feeling by adding a normative element." In other words, needs do not exist as an objective fact out there in communities. Rather, they are actively constructed, and it is argued that professionals retain power and control through the act of creating needs:

> "Indeed, it is possible to see 'meeting needs' as an ideological statement
> – a legitimation of their (professionals') practice, the protection of their
> areas of work and expertise, which must be understood in terms of the
> development of professionalism . . ." (Armstrong, 1982, p. 30).

The issue of assessing needs is discussed further in Chapter 11.

Community development strategies have been effective in highlighting women's health issues. Most community development work has been undertaken with women, and has led to innovative approaches towards major health education topics such as smoking, diet and exercise, as well as identifying a range of other health concerns. However, it has also been argued that, in general, community development has not recognized or challenged gender inequalities (Hanmer 1991). Community development focuses on class inequalities and interests, and tends to overlook gender divisions and conflicts. For example, communities tend to be defined by socio-economic indicators, such as the unemployment rate or the percentage of the population dependent on benefits. Although women are frequently targeted, gender inequalities are often considered secondary to class or ethnic inequalities. The implications of community health projects in terms of maintaining and reinforcing women's role as unpaid carers is generally overlooked (Rose, 1990). Campbell (1993) argues that this focus on economic determinants of health has meant that community development activists have colluded with ". . . men's politics masquerading as class politics . . . organized not only at the expense of women, but to the exclusion of women" (Campbell, 1993, p.231).

Dilemmas in community development practice

The question of whether the community development worker is promoting revolution or supporting the *status quo* is at the root of much of the ambiguity surrounding practice. Common dilemmas facing the community development worker relate to funding, accountability, acceptability, the role of the professional and evaluation.

Funding

Most community development projects are funded by statutory agencies, such as health and education authorities, sometimes in partnership, through joint funding. Other projects which might come under the label community development belong in the voluntary sector, and are funded from a variety of sources including direct Government grants and independent fund-raising. Most community development work is funded in the short term only. Lack of security and the impossibility of guaranteeing an input in the long term increases the problems of planning and evaluating such work. Insecure funding arrangements can also subvert a project's focus, leading workers to spend time fund-raising instead of working around defined issues.

Accountability

All community development workers have a dual accountability: to their employers and to their communities. Funding agencies naturally require projects to be accountable, and this can lead to problems where the priorities of the community and the agency are not the same. For example, Zutshi (1989) gives an account of Bristol's Inner City Health Project which points to the discrepancy between the priorities agreed by the health authority and those identified by the community. The health authority identified four main areas of concern:

    Child health and parenting
    Older people
    Mental health
 — Services for ethnic minorities.

The community identified four different priorities:

    Developing anti-racist strategies within the health services and the community
    Building community health organizations
    Developing community and user representation in the health service
    Raising awareness of health as an issue.

Attempts were made to get the health authority to agree the community's priorities. The balance must be in favour of the community; otherwise, the project is outreach under another name.

Acceptability

Employing authorities often view community development as not quite respectable. Community development may be seen as absorbing unacceptably large amounts of time and resources for dubious results. Community development tends to focus on small numbers of people whereas employers tend to be responsible for large populations. For these reasons, community development may be pursued without producing "visible" results. The long-term nature and diffuse outcomes of community development are at odds with the organizational need to allocate resources on the basis of demonstrable results.

Issues which are raised through a community development approach (such as discrimination in service provision) may be unacceptable to employing authorities. By allying themselves with dissent, the health promoter may be seen as betraying the organization.

The community development worker may also find they need to establish and negotiate their role before they are accepted by a community. Disadvantaged communities are targeted by professionals in many different ways, and sometimes these have negative results. Relationships of trust may need to be created before any other work can take place.

Role of the professional

Community development also poses problems for workers whose primary training lies in other areas.

A health visitor wishes to adopt a community development approach in her work. She has identified setting up a post-natal mums group as an appropriate project.

■ What arguments might she use in favour of this kind of work?
■ What arguments might her manager use against it?

The health visitor might argue that such work is important for health because it increases self-esteem, autonomy and confidence, and a sense of belonging. She could argue that such work is effective. For example, post-natal networking amongst mothers could prove effective in reducing psychiatric illness amongst this client group (Brown and Harris, 1978). The health visitor might also argue that time spent on setting up the group will reduce claims on her time in future, and is therefore a cost-effective option.

The health visitor's manager might respond that there is not enough time to carry out such work. Full caseloads and many other priority claims (such as visiting all new mothers and carrying out child development check-ups) mean there is no spare time available for other activities. The manager might also argue that such activities need to be thoroughly evaluated and of proven effectiveness before resources can be committed.

Problems may arise from the different kind of client/worker relationship envisaged in professional training and community development work. Professional workers are taught a particular area of expertise and tend to assume that they know what is best for their clients. They may be sensitive to individual circumstances but the secondary socialization encountered during professional training reinforces the notion of expertise.

Sociologists argue that professional culture is actually an occupational strategy designed to increase the status and rewards of the professional group (Freidson, 1986; Johnson, 1972). By acquiring professional jargon, expertise and qualifications, the professional can justify their right to practice and defend their area of work.

By contrast, community development workers see their role as that of catalyst and facilitator rather than expert. Their task is to enable a community to express its needs, and support the community in meeting those needs themselves. This requires a different worker/client relationship, based on egalitarianism and the sharing of knowledge. For professionals, whose identity is bound up in their work role, this can be a difficult switch to make.

The skills involved in community work also tend to be different to those acquired in professional training (unless this includes community development). Key skills concern process rather than content and include:

- Organizational skills, e.g. developing appropriate management structures such as management committees or steering groups
- Communication skills, e.g. consultation and communication with a variety of groups including community groups, funding agency and co-workers
- Evaluation skills, e.g. monitoring the impact of interventions and self evaluation.

■ Which of these skills are covered in your professional training?
■ How much time is devoted to these areas compared to other areas in the curriculum?
■ Do you think your professional training has equipped you to practise community development?

Evaluation

Evaluating the impact of community development work raises many questions which are discussed in greater detail in Chapter 14. What is impressive is the positive feedback from communities and workers who have been involved in community development around health issues. This is a consistent finding from many different projects, although the local scale of such work means such findings are not easily disseminated to a broader audience. To take just one example, a report of the Hartcliffe Health and Environment

Action Group, a group based in a deprived outer city housing estate in Bristol, states that:

> "From the health education point of view, this project can be seen to be instrumental in promoting people's health. A significant number of those involved would, in all probability, never otherwise have had access to information about health, health services and the support and opportunity for personal growth which has evidently been presented through their participation in this group" (Roberts, 1992, p.54).

This is typical of the enthusiasm many workers feel, which is itself a reflection of the feedback they receive from the people involved. A member of the Hartcliffe group puts it succinctly: "I don't feel like a spectator now" (Roberts, 1992, p. 37). However, these kinds of outcomes are difficult to express concisely, or to put in quantitative terms.

Despite these difficulties, it is important to evaluate community development. Ongoing or formative evaluation provides a means for results and outcomes to be fed back into a project, allowing it to be modified if necessary. Evaluation of a wide range of objectives is needed to assess the full impact of a project. Project outcomes may include changes in service provision, increased community networking, putting health on the community agenda, and increased feelings of autonomy and self-esteem.

 In 1987 the Bristol Inner City Health Project appointed an evaluation and research worker who used a variety of means to evaluate the project. These included:

- Detailed evaluation of pilot schemes and demonstration projects using
  - Interviews with workers and managers to define their objectives for evaluation
- Recording origins and development of initiatives
- Building monitoring and assessment tools into each initiative
- Health profile of the project area
- Review of staff self-evaluations
- Charting project development overall.

Conclusion

Community development does not fit tidily into most health promoters' working lives. In contrast to how most health promotion workers have been trained, community development relies upon a different set of assumptions about the nature of health and a different set of skills. This can make it a problematic activity to undertake. However, practitioners who have espoused community development are enthusiastic about its potential and outcomes. It is claimed to be the most ethical and effective form of health promotion, and one which makes a real impact on people's lives.

"What (inner city community health projects) are doing is creating a climate in which some of the most oppressed and deprived sections of our urban communities can find a voice with which to challenge the forces which both determine their health and control the quantity and quality of health services to which they have access" (Rosenthal, 1983).

Community development does appear to address many of the problems inherent in more traditional forms of health promotion. It avoids victim-blaming, addresses structural causes of inequalities in health, and seeks to empower people. This goes some way to explain its popularity with health promoters.

Community development has been endorsed at both the international level, by various WHO declarations, and at the local level, by project workers. It is not such a popular option at the middle level of large scale organizations, including the NHS. This is in part due to the practical difficulties of implementation and evaluation. However, there are also ideological conflicts if community development is to be practised within the NHS. It has been stated that community development represents a challenge to the medical model of health and previous experience in Britain has also demonstrated that it is perceived as an overtly political strategy. The political implications of community development have been attacked from both the right and the left wings of the political spectrum. Community development has been viewed as both a subversive left-wing activity, and a subtle means of policing and controlling communities.

In 1984 the Scottish Home and Health Department set up a pilot project, initially for 2 years and later extended for a further 2 years, in a deprived housing estate on the edge of Edinburgh. A community worker was appointed to work with GPs and residents, and was based first in the GP practice and later in a school. The community worker started by identifying resources and networks in the community, and together with residents undertook a small survey on views about health. The process of doing the survey led to a women's discussion group being formed. Gradually more people contacted the project for information and advice. At the same time the worker spread news about the project among colleagues in the health, education and social services. A variety of groups was set up including an Elderly Forum, a pensioners' swimming group, a fruit and vegetable co-operative, a self-help tranquillizers group which led to a stress centre being set up, and a mothers' food and families group. The project was evaluated using a number of methods including: action research, a local health survey, the use of routine hospital statistics on service use, project workers' diaries which recorded activity and reflections, a contact list, and a quasi-controlled study of parent education.

Source: RUHBC, 1989, pp. 119–137.

Questions for further discussion

■ Would you consider adopting a community development approach in your work?

■ Do you think community development has advantages over other health promotion strategies?

Summary

This chapter has examined the history and theoretical underpinnings of community development as an approach to health promotion. We have seen that community development is often viewed by workers as the most ethical and effective means of promoting health. At the same time, its practice poses dilemmas for the health promoter and its evaluation is fraught with problems. However, we would argue that the reasons put forward for the privileged position of community development are sound. Practical difficulties should not obstruct the continuing development and spread of this health promotion strategy. On the contrary, what is needed is a more open outlook from statutory organizations, and a willingness to experiment with this kind of strategy.

Further reading

Open University Health Education Unit (1991) *Community Development and Health Education*, Vol. 1, Milton Keynes, Open University Press.

This book includes a useful introduction to community development in health education and eight illustrative case studies. Issues concerning the evaluation of community development interventions are discussed.

Open University Health Education Unit (1991) *"Roots and branches": Papers from the OU/HEA 1990 Winter School on Community Development and Health*, Milton Keynes, Open University Press.

A useful collection of papers examining the theoretical roots of the community health movement and dilemmas in practice.

Smithies J and Adams L (1990) *Community Participation in Health Promotion*, London, HEA.

A brief and clear summary of different British community health promotion projects. Includes a useful glossary of key terms.

References

Armstrong P (1982) "The myth of meeting needs in adult education and community development", *Critical Social Policy*, 2 (2), 24–37.

Barclay Report on Social Work (1982). National Institute for Social Work. *Social Workers: Their Role and Tasks*, London, Bedford Square Press.

Brown G and Harris T (1978) *The Social Origins of Depression*, London, Tavistock.

Campbell B (1993) *Goliath: Britain's Dangerous Places*, London, Methuen.

Community Health Initiatives Resource Unity/London Community Health Resource (1987) *Guide to Community Health Projects*, London, NCVO.

Coulter A (1987) "Lifestyles and social class: implications for primary care", *Journal of the Royal College of General Practitioners*, **37**, 533–536.

Department of Health (1992) *The Health of the Nation*, London, HMSO.

Freidson E (1986) *Professional Powers: A Study of the Institutionalization of Formal Knowledge*, Chicago, University of Chicago Press.

Freire P (1972) *Pedagogy of the Oppressed*, Harmondsworth, Penguin.

Gatherer A *et al.* (1979) *Is Health Education Effective?* London, Health Education Council Monograph Services.

Green J and Chapman A (1991) "The lessons of the community development project for community development today", in Open University Health Education Unit (1991) *'Roots and Branches': Papers from the OU/HEA 1990 Winter School on Community Development and Health*, Milton Keynes, Open University Press.

Green LW and Raeburn J (1990) "Community wide change: Theory and practice", in N Bracht (ed.) *Health Promotion at the Community Level*, California, Sage.

Hanmer J (1991) "The influence of feminism on community development and health", in Open University Health Education Unit (1991) *'Roots and Branches': Papers from the OU/HEA 1990 Winter School on Community Development and Health*, Milton Keynes, Open University Press.

Health Education Authority (1987) Leaflet on community development.

Health Education Authority (1991) *Strategic Plan*. London, HEA.

Johnson T (1972) *Professions and Power*, London, Macmillan.

Jones J (1991) "Community development and health education: concepts and philosophy", in Open University Health Education Unit, *Community Development and Health Education*, Vol.1, Milton Keynes, Open University Press.

Mitchell J (1984) *What is to be Done about Health and Illness?* London, Pluto Press.

Research Unit in Health and Behaviour Change (1989) *Changing the Public Health*, Chichester, Wiley.

Rifkin SB (1990) *Community Participation in Maternal and Child health/family planning programmes*, Geneva, WHO.

Roberts SE (1990) *"We live there . . . we should know". A Report of Local Health Needs in Hartcliffe*, Bristol and Weston Health Promotion Department.

Roberts SE (1992) *Healthy Participation: An Evaluative Study of the Hartcliffe Health and Environment Action Group, a Community Development Project in Bristol*, unpublished dissertation.

Rose H (1990) "Activists, gender and the community health movement", *Health Promotion International*, **5**, 209–218.

Rosenthal H (1983) "Neighbourhood health projects – some new approaches to health and community work in some parts of the United Kingdom", *Community Development Journal*, **18**, 120–130.

Ross M (1955) *Community Organisation: Theories and Principles*, New York, Harper and Brothers.

Smithies J and Adams L (1990) *Community Participation in Health Promotion*, London, HEA.

Trojan A, Hildebrandt H, Deneke C and Faltis M (1991) "The role of community groups and voluntary organizations in health promotion", in Badura B and Kickbusch I (eds) *Health Promotion Research: Towards a New Social Epidemiology*, Copenhagen, WHO Regional Publications.

Watt A and Rodmell S (1988) "Community involvement in health promotion: Progress or panacea?", *Health Promotion*, **2**, 359–367.

World Health Organisation (1978) *Alma Ata 1978: Primary Health Care*, Geneva, WHO.

World Health Organisation (1985) *Targets for Health for All*, Copenhagen, WHO Regional Office for Europe.

World Health Organisation (1986) "The Ottawa charter for health promotion", *Health Promotion*, **1**, iii–v .

Zutshi M (1989) "Health service accountability and the dilemmas of community representation", *Radical Community Medicine*, Spring.

10 *Helping people to change*

Overview

Key points
- The role of beliefs, attitudes and values in health-related decisions
- The influence of social norms on health behaviour
- The concept of locus of control
- Health promotion strategies to change attitudes or behaviour.

Traditionally, behaviour or lifestyles have been regarded as the cause of many modern diseases. Therefore strategies for promoting health have derived from psychological theory which, by its nature, is individually oriented. In previous chapters we have argued that such an approach is unlikely to be effective unless it acknowledges the importance of a healthy environment and public policy-making. Many health promoters, however, see their role as helping people to live their lives to its best potential which may involve some change in their health behaviour. Understanding why you behave in certain ways and being enabled to change if you choose is a central principle of the self-empowerment approach to health promotion outlined in Chapter 5. This chapter explores the usefulness of social psychology which offers several theoretical models that identify the determinants of behaviour change. This can contribute to if not the prediction, then at least an understanding of how people make decisions about their health. This can be a useful tool in planning health promotion interventions. The influence of specific factors such as individual self esteem or people's perceptions of control over their lives needs to be taken into account by the health promoter in order to offer practical support and positive experiences in making choices.

Several theories have attempted to explain the influence of different variables on an individual's health related behaviour:

- The Health Belief Model (Becker, 1974)
- The Theory of Reasoned Action (Ajzen and Fishbein, 1980)
- The Health Action Model (Tones, 1987; Tones *et al.*, 1990)
- The Stages of Change Model (Prochaska and DiClemente, 1984).

This chapter explores the application of these models of behaviour change to health, and considers various strategies used to change attitudes or behaviour.

Definitions

According to social psychology theories of behaviour change, an individual's **attitude** to a specific action and their intention to adopt it is influenced by **beliefs**, **motivation** which comes from the person's **values**, **attitudes** and **drives or instincts**, and the influences from social norms.

A belief represents the information a person has about an object or action. It links the object to some attribute. For example, a person believes that potatoes (object) are fattening (an attribute). Theories of health-related behaviour change are based on the idea that an individual's behaviour will be based on their beliefs. In this example, the person will cut down on potatoes if they wish to lose weight. If this person is encouraged to believe that potatoes are not fattening but a useful bulk food, then they may include them in their diet. In other words, that information can influence beliefs which will then, in turn, influence behaviour. Of course, behaviour change is never quite as simple as that. Information alone is neither necessary nor sufficient for behaviour change. The health risks of smoking are well known and yet over 30% population continue to smoke.

Values These are acquired through socialization and are those emotionally charged beliefs which make up what a person thinks is important. A person's values will influence a whole range of feelings about family, friendships, career and so on. For example, values relating to sex and gender give rise to a number of attitudes towards motherhood, employment of women, body image and sexuality.

Attitudes These are more specific than values and describe relatively stable feelings towards particular issues. There is no clear association between a person's attitudes and their behaviour. Sometimes changing attitudes may stimulate a change in behaviour and sometimes behaviour change may influence attitudes. For example, many people continue to smoke despite a negative attitude to smoking. Yet once the behaviour is stopped, they may develop vehement anti-smoking views.

There are three aspects to a person's attitudes to an issue – cognitive, affective and behavioural. The cognitive component concerns a persons's knowledge and information; the affective component concerns the feelings, emotions, likes and dislikes; the behavioural component concerns a person's skills. Attitudes can be changed by providing more or different information, or by increasing a person's skills. For example, a person's attitude towards the benefits of exercise might be influenced by providing information about different types of physical activity and their effects on the body. It might also be influenced by improved performance which motivates the person and encourages them to think of exercise as enjoyable.

Drives The term "drive" is used in the Health Action Model (Tones, 1987) to describe strong motivating factors such as hunger, thirst, sex and pain. It is also used to describe motivations which can become drives such as addiction. Some studies suggest that addiction is the consequence of frequently repeated acts which become a habit and its base is a psychological fear of withdrawal (Davies, 1992). Social learning theory (Bandura, 1977) uses the term "instinct" to describe behaviours which are not learned but are present at birth. Instincts can override attitudes and beliefs. Hunger, for example, can easily override a person's favourable attitude and intention to diet.

The theoretical models which we shall now consider reflect the complexity of the relationship between behaviour and beliefs, social norms and the individual's motivation to change. They try to unpick the relative importance of these factors, recognizing that what people say is not necessarily a guide to what they will do, and that there are numerous antecedent and situational variables.

The Health Belief Model

The Health Belief Model is probably the best-known theoretical model highlighting the function of beliefs in decision making. (see Figure 10.1). This model, originally proposed by Rosenstock (1966) and modified by Becker (1974) has been used to predict protective health behaviour, such as screening or vaccination uptake and compliance with medical advice (e.g. Gillam, 1991). The model suggests that whether or not a person changes their behaviour will be influenced by an evaluation of its feasibility and its benefits weighed against its costs. In other words, a person considering changing their behaviour engages in a cost/benefit or utility analysis with themselves. This may include their beliefs concerning the likelihood of the illness or injury happening to them (their susceptibility); the severity of the illness or injury; and the efficacy of the action and whether it will have some personal benefit, or how likely it is to protect the person from the illness or injury. The Health Belief Model has been expanded to include Bandura's (1977) concept of self-efficacy. It suggests that an individual must believe they are capable of carrying out the intended behaviour. For a behavioural change to take place, an individual:

■ Must have an incentive to change
■ Feel threatened by their current behaviour

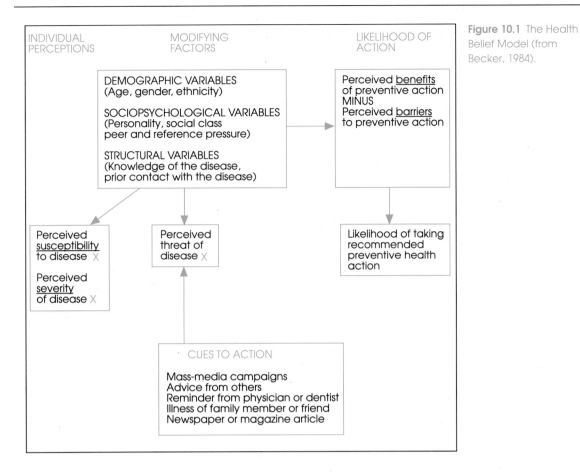

Figure 10.1 The Health Belief Model (from Becker, 1984).

■ Feel a change would be beneficial in some way and have few adverse consequences
■ Must feel competent to carry out the change.

? **Consider the following situation and then try to apply the Health Belief Model to see if you can predict how the woman might respond.**

A mother of three children under five receives a card from her GP informing her that her youngest child should receive a Hib injection to protect him from meningitis. The woman works at a local factory as an hourly paid packer. Her mother cares for the children whilst she is at work, but has no transport.

If we are to use the Health Belief Model as a model for predicting health behaviour, we would see the mother as a rational problem solver who would not only be aware of the causes of Hib meningitis but also the risks of contracting it (the child's susceptibility and severity). We would assume that the mother would have been made aware of the efficacy of the vaccine and be aware of its protection against one type of meningitis only (*Haemophilus influenzae* B). She would also be aware of any possible side effects or contraindications. If the mother has had previous children vaccinated with no adverse effects or had this child or other children immunized against other diseases, she is more likely to view this vaccination favourably and have confidence in its effectiveness. In using this model as a predictor of behaviour, we need to take into account the perceived barriers and costs to taking this action. The mother would need to ask her own

> **(cont.)**
> mother to take the child to the doctor. The child's grandmother may be unwilling or unable to take three children on public transport. Or the mother would have to take time off work with consequent loss of earnings.

Most learning theories are based on the premise that people's behaviour is guided by consequences. If these are positive or deemed to be positive, then the person is more likely to engage in that behaviour. These explanations which see behaviour as a simple response to positive or negative rewards do not seem to account for the persistence of health behaviours which have apparently negative consequences, such as smoking or drinking and driving. Obviously short-term gratification is a greater incentive than possible long-term harm.

Becker suggests that an individual is influenced by how vulnerable they perceive themselves to be to an illness, injury or danger (their **susceptibility**) and how serious they consider it to be (**severity**). People's perception and assessment of risk is central to the application of this model. Three factors appear to affect an individual's perception of risk: personal experience; ability to control the situation; and a kind of general feeling that "the illness or danger is thoroughly nasty and able to kill easily" (British Medical Association, 1987). However, in many situations people have an unrealistic optimism that "it won't happen to me".

Consideration of these variables in relation to AIDS shows the difficulties faced by AIDS educators. Many heterosexual people have an "illusion of invulnerability" (Phillips, 1993), and do not make a realistic assessment of personal risk because the social representation of AIDS is of a disease associated with gay men and injecting drug users. In a study of young people, Clift and colleagues (Clift *et al.*, 1989) found that students estimated their own risk of HIV infection to be less than their peers. In the absence of perceived risk, the perceived costs of using a condom – loss of pleasure, expense, interruption of lovemaking – may be seen as greater than any benefits.

Since beliefs may be affected by experience, direct contact with those who have a condition can powerfully affect attitudes exposing stereotypes and prejudice. For example, contact with a person who is HIV positive or who is living with AIDS can change beliefs about the fatality of the disease, and about whom is affected and how.

Those who work with young people find perceptions of risk are very different. Risk-taking is an important task of adolescence and part of separation from family. It is hard for young people to appreciate the long-term effects of, for example, smoking when 25 can seem old!

Many health education campaigns have attempted to motivate

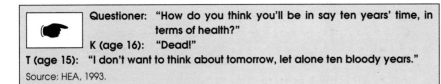

Questioner: "How do you think you'll be in say ten years' time, in terms of health?"

K (age 16): "Dead!"

T (age 15): "I don't want to think about tomorrow, let alone ten bloody years."

Source: HEA, 1993.

people to change their behaviour through fear or guilt. Drink–drive campaigns at Christmas show the devastating effects on families of road accident fatalities; smoking prevention posters urge parents not to "teach your children how to smoke". Although fear can encourage a negative attitude and even an intention to change, such feelings tend to disappear over time and when faced with a real decision-making situation. The evaluation of an extensive campaign in the mid-1980s on the dangers of drugtaking, showed it increased awareness but did not change attitudes or reduce the risk of experimentation (Dorn, 1986). Amongst non-users attitudes to heroin hardened but those who knew drug users and were therefore, most at risk, were less likely to say heroin was more dangerous than cannabis. The emotional appeal of dire portrayals (see Figure 10.2) coupled with increased mentions of drugs led to increased interest but young people tended to disregard the health message, feeling that the risks were exaggerated when their peers appeared to enjoy drugs without harmful effects. This campaign instead of frightening young people attracted them. The threat of danger and degradation seemed exciting.

The Health Belief Model suggests that people need to have some kind of cue to take action to change a behaviour or make a health-related decision. The issue needs to become salient or relevant. The cue could be noticing a change in one's internal state or appearance. For example, a pregnant woman stops smoking when she feels the baby move. It could be an external trigger, such as a change in circumstance like a job, or change in income, or the death or illness of someone close. It could be a comment from a "significant other" or a newspaper article. Health care workers can be significant others. For example, GPs' advice is taken seriously. The GP has expertise, is trustworthy and has authority, leading the patient to desire to comply. The effects of persuasive communications on attitudes is discussed more fully in Chapter 13 in the section on mass media.

? Considerable changes in sexual behaviour have taken place among gay and bisexual men in response to AIDS. However, there is a high incidence of homosexually active men engaging in what is known to be a potentially risky sexual activity, unprotected receptive anal sex.

- Consider how the Health Belief Model could be used to explain this health behaviour.
- What reasons could you offer for individuals not carrying out their intentions to act in ways that are perceived as beneficial?

Figure 10.2 "Heroin screws you up" poster.

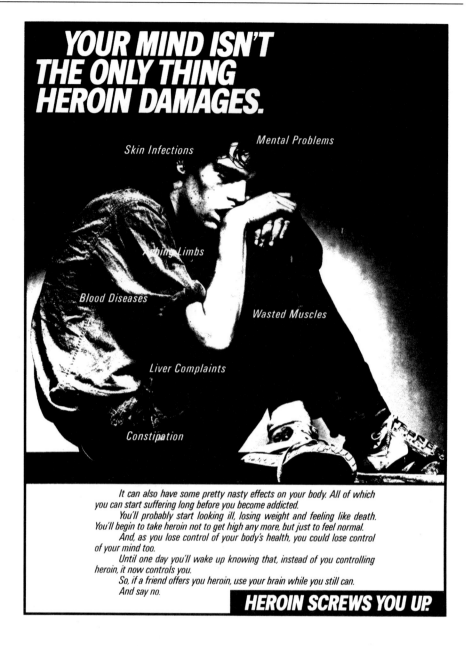

The Health Belief Model has been widely criticized. Some of these criticisms relate to its lack of weighting for different factors – all cues to preventive action, for example, are seen as equally salient. Stainton Rogers offers a strong critique of psychological models which attempt to explain complex behaviour as assuming "the whole is no more than the (albeit complex) 'sum of the parts'; that actions are informed and chosen via analysis of a set of conceptual components isolated from one another. They have no place for the kinds of interwoven, articulated arguments and stories which form the fabric of conversation and of media messages" (Stainton Rogers, 1993, p. 55).

Theory of Reasoned Action

According to the Theory of Reasoned Action (Ajzen and Fishbein, 1980), a person's behaviour can be predicted by their intentions. Intention is, in turn, a function of attitude towards that behaviour. A person's attitude will be a result of their perceived consequences of the behaviour and their perception about what others expect them to do (subjective norms). These two influences on attitudes combine to form an intention. The main task is to discover the relative influence of the attitude to the act and the subjective norm component.

> Consider the example of smoking behaviour.
>
> A person may have certain feelings about smoking based on their experience and whether their family and friends smoke. Women may believe that smoking will keep down their weight. The Theory of Reasoned Action includes personality traits as an influence on health behaviour, and therefore we might consider the person's attitude to risk-taking and authority. Alongside these attitudes will be those of significant others and whether the individual wishes to comply with them. What does the person's mother think about smoking? Or their GP?
>
> The individual will then consider the relative importance of these attitudinal and normative components and this will then result in an intention to smoke – or to stop smoking. For example, concern about how the outside world sees you may be more important than the feelings of enjoyment, relaxation or coping that derive from smoking.

Ajzen and Fishbein (1985) acknowledge that people do not necessarily behave consistently with their intentions. The ability to predict behaviour will be influenced by the stability of a person's belief. Stability is determined by strength of belief, how long it has been held, whether it is reinforced by other groups to which the individual belongs, whether it is related to and integrated with other attitudes and beliefs, and how clear or structured it is.

The Theory of Reasoned Action differs from the Health Belief Model in that it suggests that people's perceptions of the attitudes of others towards the behaviour could be a powerful influence. Figure 10.3 shows the significance of this factor in the Theory of Reasoned Action. The motivation to comply with perceived social pressure from "significant others" could cause a person to behave in a way that they believe these other people or groups would think is right. The influence of so-called peer group pressure (even if it does not amount to pressure) can be very powerful within a

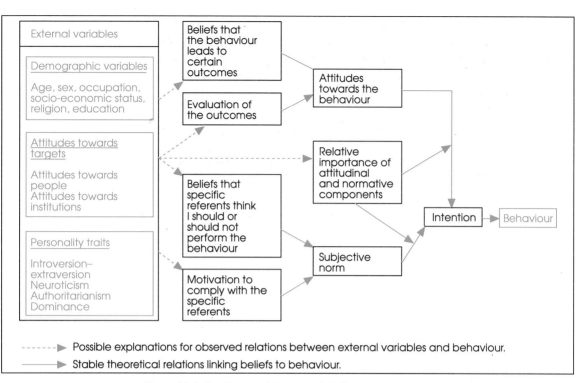

Figure 10.3 The Theory of Reasoned Action (from Azjen and Fishbein, in: *Understanding Attitudes and Predicting Social Behavior*, Azjen and Fishbein (Eds), © 1990, pp. 5–11. Reprinted by permission of Prentice-Hall, Inc., Englewood Cliffs, NJ).

small group if the individual values membership of that group or wants to belong to it.

> **?** **Think of an occasion where social norms have influenced a health-related decision on your part. What was the most powerful aspect of this influence? Consider the following examples of conformity to social norms.**
>
> ■ An example of public acceptance and private autonomy: "Ann goes on holiday with a group of friends. On the first evening it becomes apparent that no one smokes. Rather than ask if anyone minds if she does, Ann retires early to bed and has a solitary cigarette".
>
> ■ An example of temporary acceptance of group mores: "Bill works in a predominantly male office. At the end of the day, five or six people adjourn to a local bar. The men are eager to establish themselves by buying a round of drinks. Bill waits until everyone has finished before offering to buy a round by which time someone else has got to the bar. Bill usually only drinks one pint of beer but he stays until everyone has bought a round – six pints.

There are occasions when there is inconsistency in a person's beliefs. This has been termed "cognitive dissonance" by Festinger (1957). For example, a nurse who smokes and who is educating a patient recovering from a heart attack is faced with a psychological dilemma: does she follow her professional training or does she acknowledge her personal need and desire to smoke? Pressure builds up on the nurse to reconcile this unpleasant state of affairs either by changing her attitude to smoking or by changing her attitude to patient education.

 Consider the example of Catherine who is told by her teacher that she is a talented athlete. Her friends believe exercise is not "cool" and try to avoid it as much as possible. Catherine enjoys sport, and feels fitter and exhilarated after exercise. She is thus in a state of tension. She could:

■ Change her attitude to exercise and agree with her friends that it is not worth the bother
■ Lose her favourable attitude to her teacher and feel her teacher is only flattering her
■ Change her attitude to her friends and accept that they are merely carrying out their choice.

The role of modelling has been particularly important in health promotion. Concern has been expressed that indirect modelling of behaviour may come from watching television. For example, people on television are able to drink heavily without any apparent ill effects (Hansen, 1986). Direct modelling is sometimes assumed to be less influential, but models who have status and credibility, such as musicians and people in sport have been used to present health promotion messages. If people are influenced by role models, then health promoters may themselves be taken as exemplars. Ewles and Simnett (1992) raise concern over the health promoter whose lifestyle is at odds with the health-promoting ways they advocate.

Some health education programmes have used peer group leaders to influence behaviour such as "Smoking and Me" or the MESMAC (Men Who Have Sex With Men) project. The rationale is that "significant others" have credibility, are able to communicate in appropriate ways and are models to follow, although doubts may be expressed about the skills and information that peer educators possess.

Social norms include peer group or family beliefs, but also what are perceived to be "general" norms as conveyed by, for example, the mass media. What is important is what the individual believes other people do, not the actual extent of the activity. The Joint Breastfeeding Initiative has, for example, complained that the low number of young mothers who choose to breast feed is partly due to their perception that other women bottle feed. The World Health Organisation have identified the importance of formal and informal social networks to support individuals and give people assistance in the pursuit of health (WHO, 1986). Group techniques, such as those used by Alcoholics Anonymous, appear to have some success by getting clients to identify with the group through personal testimony and a public commitment, which encourages the group to then provide support for each other.

The Theory of Reasoned Action suggests that behaviour change is a function of:

- Beliefs about the consequences of the behaviour
- Evaluation of the importance of the outcome
- The expectations of significant others
- A motivation to conform.

The Health Action Model

The Health Action Model (Figure 10.4) is less well known but is highlighted in some health promotion literature. It is included here because it identifies self-esteem to be a key component in the motivation system (Tones, 1987; Tones *et al.*, 1990). The motivation system describes a complex of affective elements including a person's values, drives and self esteem. The centrality of the motivation system differentiates this model from the Health Belief Model and the Theory of Reasoned Action.

The ways in which individuals view themselves will be a major influence on their readiness to take a health decision. Self-esteem means the evaluation a person makes of him- or herself – a personal judgement of worth expressed in the attitudes a person holds towards themselves. So we talk of high or low self-esteem in the sense of feeling more or less worthwhile and valued. Self-concept is a global term which refers to all those beliefs which people have about themselves – about their abilities and their attributes. It includes ideas about appearance, intelligence and physical skills. It is built and modified through our perceptions of the way other people behave towards us, how we are accepted and affirmed, or rejected and criticized. It will thus also derive from having a network of social support.

The development of self-concept and self-esteem has been at the centre of work in health education and promotion. It is assumed that a person with high self-esteem is likely to feel confident about themselves and have social and life skills which will enhance their feelings of personal efficacy. Because of their feelings of personal effectiveness, the person's self-esteem is enhanced.

Many health education programmes particularly those targeted at young people, have been based on the premise that there is a relationship between self-esteem and health behaviour (Health

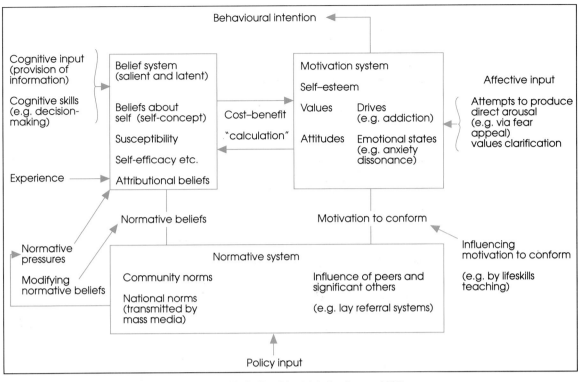

Figure 10.4 Health promotion and the Health Action Model (after Tones, 1987).

Education Council, 1983). Those who engage in health-damaging behaviour such as drug taking are thought to have low self-esteem reinforced by poor social relationships. However, there is an argument that the majority of young people who use drugs casually are more confident and more risk-taking and may, according to all attitude measures, have higher self-esteem (Chapman, 1992).

Drug education programmes have focused on boosting self-esteem by equipping young people with efficacy skills like resisting peer group pressure and self-awareness. However, what takes place in a classroom may bear little relation to the social context in which drug use takes place. The advertising agency who tested the Government drug education commercials in 1986 acknowledge this in their report:

"It is our impression that convictions about how evil/stupid/destructive heroin is fall away with surprising ease when apparently contradicted by the example of a friend. A friendly offer and easy accessibility seem to cut heroin down to size and the dangers with it" (Dorn, 1986).

The ways in which this educational approach has been extended in the self-empowerment model of health promotion is described in Chapter 5. Providing understanding, clarifying values, practising decision making and assertiveness skills may help the individual towards specific health-related goals. The methods used in these approaches are participative. The learner is actively involved and can develop an understanding, through various educational strategies, such as role play, of the ways in which different factors affect their decisions. Education does not, of course, modify the environment and, as we saw in Chapter 5, self-empowerment in health promotion would take a wider role, enabling people to work together to influence services and policy in their community.

> **?**
>
> **There has been a great deal of work in sports education on building behaviour and attitude patterns which will maintain a commitment to exercise (e.g. Biddle, 1987). Part of this concerns an individual's confidence to participate in physical activity which can be damaged by competition, an overemphasis on skill or ability comparisons.**
>
> Consider what might influence an individual's belief that they can carry out an exercise programme and then read the following list of factors:
>
> ■ Successful performance
> ■ Vicarious experience (observing those who are similar to themselves, not high level sports stars)
> ■ Persuasion by a credible source
> ■ Positive attributions, such as fitness and weight loss
> ■ Physiological arousal.

The notion of perceived control as a mediating factor in behaviour has received a great deal of attention since its original development as part of social learning theory by Rotter (1954). Social learning theory suggests that the ways in which people explain the things that happen to them is a product of their childhood experiences. Those who are rewarded for their successes, and punished consistently and fairly will come to believe that they are in control of their lives, and will develop a realistic assessment of their own capabilities.

Control in the context of health can be understood in terms of:

■ Internal locus of control (the extent to which a person believes that they are responsible for their own health).

Those with an external locus of control believe their actions are limited by:

■ Powerful others
■ Chance, fate or luck.

Research has focused on categorizing attitudes to health by using a locus of control measure such as a multiple choice inventory. It has been assumed that those who have a strong internal locus of control will see themselves as more coping, and more able to act decisively and capably and will be those people who undertake preventive health actions or change to more healthy behaviours. So far it has generally been found that there is only a weak relationship between feelings of control and specific behaviours, although associations have been found with smoking cessation and weight loss and the propensity to use preventive medical services (Wallston *et al.*, 1978). Indeed a lifestyle survey of 9000 adults found that "unhealthy" kinds of behaviour are more likely to be associated with an internal locus of control (Blaxter *et al.*, 1990). At the same time those who recorded positive or responsible attitudes to health were also more likely to have a high locus of control. This confirms the argument earlier in this chapter that specific behaviour cannot necessarily be predicted from attitudes.

Stainton Rogers has written a highly critical account of the work on locus of control suggesting that most research has only established self-evident differences between groups of people which had little to do with their health beliefs. People who register as "externals" on the multi-dimensional health locus of control scale are those with lower levels of education, and of lower socio-economic class – in other words, people who have every reason to believe that they do not have much control over their lives or health status (Stainton Rogers, 1993).

The Stages of Change Model

Although it may seem self-evident to the health promoter that a change in health behaviour would be beneficial for a client, it is often very difficult to encourage such changes and clients may not respond to advice.

The work of Prochaska and DiClemente (1984) in developing a stage model of behaviour acquisition is important in showing that any change we make is not an ending but one of a whole series. Their work has been in encouraging change in addictive behaviours, although the model can be used to show that most people go through a number of stages when trying to change or acquire behaviours. Figure 10.5 illustrates this process with the following stages identified:

Precontemplation. The person has not considered changing their lifestyle or become aware of any potential risks in their health behaviour.

Contemplation. Although the individual is aware of the benefits of change, they are not yet ready and may be seeking information or help to make that decision. This stage may last a short while or several years.

Preparing to change. When the perceived benefits seem to outweigh the costs and when the change seems possible as well as worthwhile, the individual may be ready to change, perhaps seeking some extra support.

Figure 10.5 The Stages of
Change Model (after
Prochaska and
DiClemente, 1984).

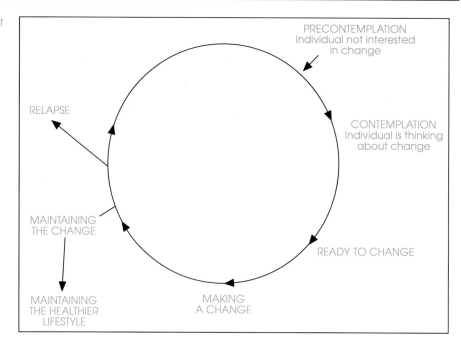

Making the change. The early days of change require positive decisions by the individual to do things differently. A clear goal, a realistic plan, support and rewards are features of this stage.

Maintenance. The new behaviour is sustained and the person moves into a healthier lifestyle.

Prochaska *et al.* (1992) argue that whilst few people go through each stage in an orderly way, they will go through each stage. This has proved helpful for many health care workers who find it reassuring that a "relapse" on the part of their clients is not a failure, but that the individual can go both backwards and forwards through a series of cycles of change – like a revolving door. Thus a smoker may stop smoking many times before finally giving up completely. Nevertheless the client is still aware of the benefits of giving up smoking and the health care worker may be able to focus on such small changes, which can provide themselves and their client with a sense of achievement and identifiable progress.

Whilst individuals may not have an awareness of contemplating, actioning and maintaining change, the intention will be based on an individual deciding it is in their best interests to change. The key to successful interventions then is for a client to be motivated. Health promoters must bear in mind that their clients may not share their perceptions about the worth of a particular behaviour. However, evidence from a study of nurses helping people to stop smoking, showed that where clients are strongly involved in the planning process they are more likely to be motivated (MacLeod Clark and Dines, 1993).

Identifying a precontemplative stage is important because it reminds the health care worker to be aware that a client is not ready to change and therefore their work should focus on other issues, perhaps ensuring a "safer" lifestyle. For example, an injecting drug user who chooses to continue to use drugs may be advised to use a needle exchange scheme.

The Stages of Change model differs from the other models of behaviour change described in this chapter because it is principally about how people change and not why people do not change. It has been criticized for suggesting that there are specific interventions that can be matched with each stage (Davidson, 1992). For the health promoter, however, it offers a useful guide to behaviour change.

The prerequisites of change

A longitudinal study of working-class mothers in South Wales has shown how it is relatively easy to influence attitudes or behaviour, but difficult to sustain changes in health behaviour over a longer period (Pill, 1990). This study of self-initiated change shows the importance of precipitating life events and the minor part played by health concerns. For example, women who gave up smoking did so to save money and those who took up exercise did so to join in with their children.

The importance of considering the social context and everyday life is brought out clearly by this study which showed that eventually most women reverted to their original behaviours because of the influence of partners or children, or because it was too difficult to juggle personal and family priorities.

The evidence from people who have changed their health behaviour suggests that there are certain minimum conditions required for that change to take place (RUHBC, 1989).

1. The change must be self-initiated

Some people react adversely or wish to contain any attempt to look at their "unhealthy behaviour". To some people, their behaviour may not seem "unhealthy" at all but may constitute a clear source of well-being, its benefits far outweighing its risks. There is a clear message here for those health educators who work with individual clients and who are sometimes accused of "telling people what to do" – people will only change if they want to!

2. The behaviour must become salient

Most health-related behaviours including smoking, alcohol use, eating and exercise (or lack of it) are habitual, and built into the flow of everyday life such that the individual does not give them much thought. For a change to occur, that behaviour or habit must be called into question by some other activity or event so that the behaviour becomes "salient". For example, a smoker going to live with a non-smoker causes the smoking behaviour to be reappraised. The death of a relative from breast cancer may similarly prompt a woman to go for screening.

3. The salience of the behaviour must appear over a period of time

The habitual behaviour needs to become difficult to maintain. The new behaviour must, in turn, become part of everyday life. For example, one reason why people on diets often resume their previous eating patterns is because they are made constantly aware of the diet and it is never allowed to become a habit. Similarly, exercise is often not maintained because it requires effort, hence the advice to reluctant "couch potatoes" to build physical activity into their daily life by walking to work or running up stairs rather than going out to exercise at a pool or gym.

4. The behaviour is not part of the individual's coping strategies

People have various sources of comfort and solace, and will resist change to these behaviours. It is sometimes possible to enable clients to identify alternative coping strategies. For example, a person who eats chocolate when depressed may be encouraged to become physiologically aroused by taking up jogging.

5. The individual's life should not be problematic or uncertain

There is a limit to a person's capacity to adapt and change. For example, those living on low incomes will be stretched by coping with poverty and its uncertainties. Having to make changes in their health behaviour may be too much to expect for people whose lives are already problematic.

6. Social support is available

The presence and interest of other people provides reinforcement and keeps the behaviour salient. Changing one's behaviour can be stressful and individuals need support. The influence of peer-group pressure and support is not given sufficient weight in the various psychological theories of change. The World Health Organisation recognized the important role for the health promoter in stimulating and maintaining social supports for individuals and groups (WHO, 1986).

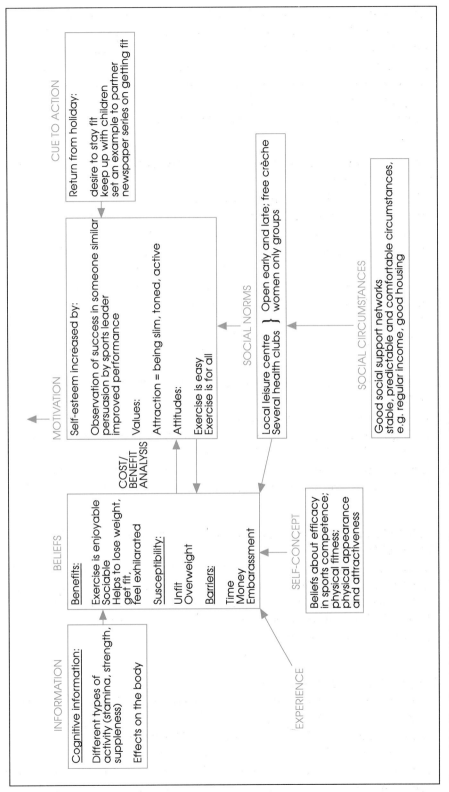

Figure 10.6 Health-related behaviour change: the example of exercise for women.

Look at Figure 10.6 which shows a diagrammatic representation of some of the influences on a person's decision to take up an exercise programme.
Think about an attempt you have made to enhance your health.

- Were you successful in the change?
- What influenced you to make the change?
- Can you identify any specific triggers that prompted you to make the change?
- How do your family and friends regard the behaviour?
- What were the costs and benefits of making the change?

Look at the list of minimum conditions above, do any of these factors help to explain your success or failure in making the health-related behaviour change?

Conclusion

The application of social psychology to health promotion has attracted criticism because it is believed that behaviour is not the most important determinant of health, and working to change attitudes and behaviour minimizes the structural inequalities which limit people's potential for health. Nevertheless behaviour change remains a feature of many approaches to health promotion and we have argued in this book that this must be accompanied by programmes which attempt to provide the environmental conditions which make the healthy choice the easier choice. The role of health education and promotion is neatly summarized by Whitehead and Tones:

> "One level involves primarily influencing beliefs (assuming that attempts to directly 'plug into' motivation by creating fear or otherwise generate emotional responses are of dubious value both ethically and in terms of effectiveness). The other level is concerned with providing the understanding and skills needed to translate intention into practice. Health education is also concerned to foster healthy public policy in order to encourage the development of a health-promoting environment that both will facilitate intentions to make healthy choices and will signal the unacceptability of unhealthy practices" (Whitehead and Tones, 1991, p.13).

What is clear from this outline of psychological theories of behaviour change is that none provides a full explanation. However, the variables identified by these models do appear in people's accounts of their health behaviour:

- Perceptions of risk and vulnerability
- Perceptions of the severity of the disease
- Perceived effectiveness of behaviour.

Whilst they may not help to predict who will adopt preventive health practices, they can help to plan programmes of education by making clear those factors which influence decisions.

 Although the efficacy of breast self-examination has been questioned, 90% of breast cancers are detected by women themselves (Faulder, 1992). There is value then in promoting early detection methods including breast awareness and mammography for those eligible. Using a model of behaviour change may help in planning programmes on beast cancer and its detection:

- Women are not well informed about the risk factors for breast cancer
- They cannot make a realistic assessment of their own susceptibility
- Personal risks tend to be overestimated which can result in fear and denial
- Women believe that most people with cancer will not be cured
- Women are not confident in their ability to detect a breast lump
- Women regard screening as an inconvenience

Source: Pitts, 1993.

Key elements in a successful campaign might be:

1. The provision of accurate information to all women
2. Information to enable individuals to identify their personal risk
3. A campaign to emphasize that the quality of living with cancer is improved with treatment even when the disease is not curable
4. Breast awareness to be taught by all health care workers
5. Improvements in the call/recall system
6. The campaign is publicized through women's networks to engender social support.

Questions for further discussion

- Do social psychology theories help you to understand the reasons why people may or may not change their health behaviour?
- What factors should health promoters take into account when helping a client to change their health behaviour?

Summary

This chapter has reviewed the role of psycho-social factors in health behaviour and discussed four theoretical models. These models have been used to explain and predict health-related decisions, such as screening or compliance to a medical regimen. All the models identify some common variables which influence the likelihood of a person adopting "healthy" behaviours: beliefs about the efficacy of the new behaviour; motivation and how much they value their health enough to change; normative pressures and the influence of significant people around them. The limitations of the role of social psychology in health promotion are outlined but it is concluded that an understanding of those factors influencing individual behaviour can help in planning appropriate health promotion interventions.

Further Reading

Bennett P and Hodgson R (1992) "Psychology and health promotion", in Bunton R and Macdonald G *Health promotion: Disciplines and Diversity*, pp. 23–42, London, Routledge.

A summary of the theories which attempt to explain the process of change in health-related behaviours. The chapter illustrates the use of psychological theories in the development of health promotion programmes.

Downie RS, Fyfe C and Tannahill A (1990) *Health Promotion: Models and Values*, Oxford, Oxford Medical Publications.

Chapters 7,8 and 9 include useful attempts to describe and define the role of health beliefs, attitudes and values.

Open University (1993) *K258 Health and Wellbeing*, Milton Keynes, Open University Press.

Part 1, Section 2 of this second-level course looks at the ways in which lay people describe their health and their accounts of personal change.

Research Unit in Health and Behavioural Change (1989),

Changing the Public Health, Chichester, Wiley.

Chapter 5 is a packed account of research findings relating to behaviour change. The chapter outlines the limitations of social psychology models and suggests its own theory of behaviour change.

Tones K, Tilford S and Keeley Robinson Y (1990) *Health Education: Effectiveness and Efficiency*, London, Chapman & Hall.

Chapter 3 provides a short but clear account of the theoretical models which seek to explain the relationship between knowledge, beliefs, attitudes, social pressures and environmental constraints. It concentrates on the Health Action Model.

References

Ajzen I and Fishbein M (1980) *Understanding Attitudes and Predicting Social Behaviour*, Englewood Cliffs, Prentice Hall.

Bandura A (1977) *Social Learning Theory*, Englewood Cliffs, Prentice Hall.

Becker MH (ed.) (1974) *The Health Belief Model and Personal Health Behaviour*, Thorofare New Jersey, Slack.

Biddle SJH (1987) *Foundations of Health-related Fitness in Physical Education*, London, Ling.

Blaxter M (1990) *Health and Lifestyles*, London, Tavistock.

British Medical Association (1987) *Living With Risk* Wiley, Chichester.

Chapman C (1992) *Drugs Issues for Schools*, Institute for the Study of Drug Dependence, London.

Clift SM, Stears D, Legg S, Memon A and Ryan L (1989) *The HIV/AIDS Education and Young People Project: Report on Phase One*, Horsham, AVERT.

Davidson R (1992) Editorial: Procahaska and DiClemente model of change, *British Journal of Addiction*, **87**, 821–822.

Davies JB (1992) *The Myth of Addiction*, Reading, Harwood.

Dorn N (1986) "Media campaigns", *Druglink*, July/August.

Ewles L and Simnett I (1992) *Promoting Health*, London, Scutari.

Faulder C (1992) "Breast awareness: what do we really mean?", *European Journal of Cancer*, **28A**, 1595–1596.

Festinger L (1957) *A Theory of Cognitive Dissonance*, University Press, Stanford

Gillam S (1991) Understanding the uptake of cervical cancer screening: the contribution of Health Belief Model, *British Journal of General Practice*, **41**, 510–513.

Hansen A (1986) "The portrayal of alcohol on television", *Health Education Journal*, **45**, 3.

Health Education Authority (1993) *The Health Action Pack*, HEA, London.

Health Education Council (1983) *My Body Project,* London, HEC.

MacLeod Clark J and Dines A (1993) "Nurses working with people who wish to stop smoking", in Dines A and Cribb A *Health Promotion: Concepts and Practice*, pp. 67–84, Oxford, Blackwell.

Phillips K (1993) "Primary prevention of AIDS", in Pitts M and Phillips K (eds) *The Psychology of Health*, London, Routledge and Kegan Paul.

Pill RM (1990) "Change and stability in health behaviour: a five year follow-up study of working-class mothers", in *Lifestyle, Health and Health Promotion*, pp. 63–79, Health Promotion Research Trust, Cambridge.

Prochaska JO and DiClemente C (1984) *The Transtheoretical Approach: Crossing Traditional Foundations of Change*, Harnewood, IL, Don Jones/Irwin.

Prochaska JO, DiClemente C and Norcross JC (1992) "In search of how people change", *American Psychologist*, **47**, 1102–1114.

Rosenstock I (1966 Why people use health services, *Millbank Memorial Fund Quarterly*, **44**, 94–121.

Rotter JB (1954) *Social Learning and Clinical Psychology*, Englewood Cliffs, Prentice Hall.

Stainton Rogers W (1993) *Explaining Health and Illness: an Exploration of Diversity*, Hemel Hempstead, Harvester.

Tones BK (1987) "Devising strategies for preventing drug misuse: the role of the Health Action Model", *Health Education Research*, **2**, 305–317.

Tones K, Tilford S and Keeley Robinson Y (1990) *Health Education; Effectiveness and Efficiency*, London, Chapman & Hall

Wallston KA, Wallston BS and DeVellis RF (1978) "Locus of control and health: a review of the literature", *Health Education Monographs*, **6**, 107–117.

Whitehead M and Tones K (1991) *Avoiding the Pitfalls*, London, HEA.

World Health Organisation (1986) "Lifestyles and health", *Social Science Medicine*, **22**, 117–124.

SECTION 3
Working for Health Promotion

This section is concerned with the implementation of health promotion. How do we assess our clients' needs? Should health promotion interventions be targeted to particular groups? What strategies have been successful and what needs to be taken into account when planning a health promotion programme? Above all, how will we know if health promotion works?

Assessing needs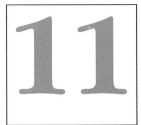

Overview

The first phase in health promotion planning is an assessment of what a client or population group needs to enable them to become more healthy. This chapter explores the concept of need and how this may be perceived differently by different groups. The purpose of Health Needs Assessment at national, regional or local level is twofold:

- to identify which improvements in health should have greatest priority
- to choose which particular groups or communities should have priority and to help in targeting interventions.

Recognition of the right to participate in defining health needs and health care was acknowledged in the 1977 WHO Alma Ata declaration and one of the underlying principles of Health For All is community participation (WHO, 1977). Consumerism is very much part of the reforms of the NHS and other public sectors that have taken place in the 1980s and 1990s. This chapter considers the ways in which individual and local health needs are assessed and applied in planning for health promotion. It should be read in conjunction with Chapter 3 which outlines the principal sources of information about health status.

Understanding health needs

What do we mean by need? The concept is so widely used: "this family needs financial assistance"; "we should give it to those who need it most"; "I need a new coat"; "I need you".

A need is something people could benefit from. It should be distinguished from a demand which is something people ask for, and supply which is what is provided. The purpose of a need must be deemed worthwhile for it to be perceived as need. For example, I need a new coat. Why? To be warm and look fashionable. Is that a worthwhile goal or is it merely that I want a new coat? Maslow's (1954) famous hierarchy of needs shows the health promoter that

How would you distinguish between a need, a want, or a demand?

203

Figure 11.1 Maslow's
hierarchy of needs (from
Oliver, 1993).

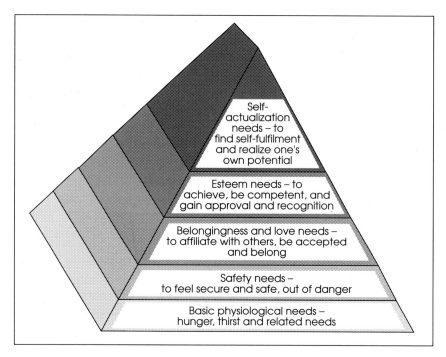

all human needs are in fact health needs (see Figure 11.1). Social
and economic conditions must first be satisfied before an individual
can personally grow and gain "self-actualization".

Concepts of need

Bradshaw (1972) in a widely used taxonomy, distinguished four
types of need: normative, felt, expressed and comparative need.

Normative needs

These are objective needs as defined by professionals. A normative
need reflects a professional judgement that a person or persons
deviates from a required standard. This may be against some
external criteria such as occupational or legal requirements. Thus
the manager of a restaurant is in need of training because s/he has
not completed a course in food hygiene. Or it may be that a person
deviates from what is defined as the range of "clinically normal".

 A Health visitor decides that, according to a growth chart, an infant
has failed to gain weight for some time and has fallen below the third
centile. She deems the infant to be in need of supplementary
feeding and suggests this is done by additional bottle feeding. Yet expectations
of child development vary according to the place and time. This infant would not
be regarded as failing to thrive in the USA or in pre-War Britain.

Normative needs are not absolute or objective "facts" – they reflect the judgement of the professional which may be different from that of their clients. Health care workers will judge a need relative to what they are able to provide. For example, a health visitor may believe there is a need for a teenage mothers' support group based on her judgement of "good standards" of parenting. But the women themselves may see their needs as the alleviation of poverty, more council housing and safe play areas.

Felt needs

Felt needs are what people really **want**. They are needs identified by clients themselves which may relate to services, information, or support which can be termed service needs. Or it may be a need, experienced subjectively, of feeling unwell according to a person's personal standards of health which can be termed a health need. Armstrong (1982) describes felt needs as "perceived needs" stemming from "within" and not ascribed from "without". Moves towards bottom-up approaches in health and welfare have meant a greater acceptance of clients' views. However, needs may be limited by the perceptions of an individual. Someone may not believe themselves to be in need simply because they do not know what is available in terms of treatment or services.

> **?**
>
> **A GP practice is aware that a lot of patients are seeking consultations for their concerns about not getting pregnant. The practice decides to hold an evening talk on preconceptual care. The talk is advertised in the surgery. No one attends.**
>
> ■ On what grounds did the practice decide there was a need?
> ■ Why did the practice decide the need was for preconceptual care?
> ■ What other needs might patients have in this area?
> ■ What other response might the practice have to this patient need?
>
> This is an example of a need identified by professionals. No consultation was involved.
> The intervention was planned in the expectation that it would result in a saving of GP time not as part of a programme to prioritize infertility. The intervention was poorly presented with no marketing, and no attempt to make it accessible for clients.

Expressed need

Expressed need arises from felt needs but is expressed in words or action – it has become a **demand**. Thus a client or group is expressing a need when they ask for help or information, or when they make use of a service. Sometimes people will use a service because it is all that is available even if it does not adequately meet needs. The best example of expressed need (and unmet demand) is the waiting list. Some needs are not expressed, perhaps because of an inability or unwillingness to articulate the need. This could be due to language difficulties or a lack of knowledge. Expressed needs should not be taken as an indicator of demand because they exclude needs which are felt but not expressed. Tudor Hart's Inverse Care Law has been of vital importance in showing that just because a service or treatment is used less it does not mean it is needed less (Tudor Hart, 1971). Those who could most benefit from a service are least likely to use it. People may express different needs, and there is a tendency to listen to those with loud and powerful voices, such as views which come from an established group or Community Health Council or views which appear to express a popular need.

> **?** The National Breast Screening Programme introduced in 1988 for all women aged 50 to 64 had a 70% take up in the year 1990/1.
>
> ■ What kind of need is the programme designed to meet?
> ■ What kind of need does the take-up rate suggest?

Comparative needs

A person or group is said to be in need if their situation, when compared with that of a similar group or individual is found "wanting" or lacking with regard to services and resources. For example, if a person with schizophrenia in District A was living in sheltered accommodation and receiving day care, but in District B this was not available, we would say schizophrenics in District B were "in need". In the NHS whilst people may be assessed to be in absolute need (normatively), in practice comparative needs assessment will often dictate whether their needs will be met. Districts may be compared on the basis of provision of services or length of waiting lists to see if the health needs of their populations are being met. This kind of analysis of need does, of course, assume that those in receipt of a service are receiving adequate provision and that a need is being satisfied.

So we can see that needs are not objective and observable entities to which we just need to match our interventions. The concept of need is a relative one and is influenced both by values and attitudes and by other agendas. Illich *et al.* (1977) have argued that the essential nature of a profession is its possession of knowledge and authority to determine what people "need". Professionals can then offer a service to meet those needs, and in so doing maintain their own status and resources.

> Consider these interventions available to women in childbirth. Has medicine created these needs or are they needed improvements in technology?

(cont.)
- **Prostaglandin to induce labour**
- **Epidural to reduce pain**
- **Electronic foetal monitoring**
- **Belt monitoring of contractions.**

At first sight, these developments may be seen as the consequence of medical advances. However, medical interventions in childbirth can also be seen as an attempt to establish doctors' control over that of midwives. The range of interventions, on the one hand, may alienate women and make childbirth an uncomfortable and distressing experience and, on the other hand, the very availability of these services may create a need for them.

Background to health needs assessment

The process of assessing needs is nothing new. As we shall see in the next chapter, understanding needs is integral to a basic process approach to planning. Needs assessment including the collection of data is the first step, from which subsequent aims will be worked out.

The NHS reforms put a new emphasis on the needs of a local population. The White Paper Working for Patients stated: "District Health Authorities will concentrate on ensuring that the health needs of the population for which they are responsible are met. . ." (Department of Health, 1989, 2.11).

The NHS defines need as the population's ability to benefit from health services which range from prevention through care and treatment to rehabilitation. This basic principle has far-reaching implications. The NHS will assess health needs and then identify actions capable of being delivered by the NHS and which will achieve "health gain". The concept of health gain includes increasing life expectancy by a reduction in premature deaths and improving well-being and quality of life. The health gain approach is seen as "Adding Years to Life and Life to Years."

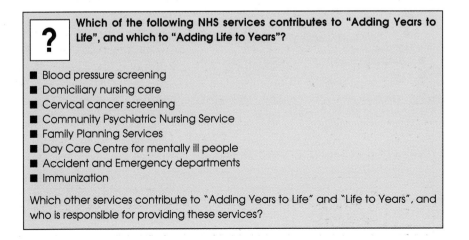

? **Which of the following NHS services contributes to "Adding Years to Life", and which to "Adding Life to Years"?**

- Blood pressure screening
- Domiciliary nursing care
- Cervical cancer screening
- Community Psychiatric Nursing Service
- Family Planning Services
- Day Care Centre for mentally ill people
- Accident and Emergency departments
- Immunization

Which other services contribute to "Adding Years to Life" and "Life to Years", and who is responsible for providing these services?

One of the major recommendations of the Acheson report (Acheson, 1988) was that Health Authorities should produce an Annual Report on the health of their population. The purpose of the report is to provide a regular epidemiological assessment of the population's health from which joint planning and policy development can be planned, and against which improvements can be measured. Whilst the moves to coordinating a health strategy are to be welcomed, there are drawbacks in allowing "epidemiology to drive the system" (Tannahill, 1992). The mortality and morbidity data tend to set the health promotion agenda and the focus for prevention. We then become concerned only with disease and people's subjective experience, and social and psychological health needs are untapped. Despite the inclusion of social indicators, health behaviour is not seen in its social context and so there is a tendency to focus on individual responsibility rather than the determinants of health.

A central feature of the national health strategy is health improvement targets and milestones which are to be achieved over a stated period of time. The Health of the Nation strategy states that both purchaser and provider services in the NHS should consult on local needs in order to set these targets for health gain and to involve users in an assessment of the services that are provided.

> "To give people an effective voice will call for a radically different approach from in the past . . . Health Authorities have a dual responsibility to ensure that the voice of local people is heard. Firstly, they need to encourage local people to be involved in the purchasing process. Secondly, they need to ensure that the providers take account of local needs in their activities" (NHS Management Executive, 1992).

The purpose of assessing health needs

1. To help in directing interventions appropriately

 A male patient who is young and fit has a heart attack. The nurse on the ward offers the patient advice on cardiac rehabilitation and information on healthy eating, exercise and safe drinking.

- Is the nurse meeting the patient's needs?
- Is health education information an appropriate intervention?

The medical and individualistic approach is adopted because it is a well understood part of the nurse's professional role. The nurse understands coronary heart disease prevention as focusing on risk factors even though they are not relevant to this situation. The patient may have other health needs such as a concern about getting back to work or when he might be sexually active again. Assessing individual health needs means starting with the patient's own concerns.

2. To identify and respond to specific needs of minority groups, communities or sections of the population whose health needs have not been fully met

> **?** A district aims to reduce mortality from coronary heart disease and stroke by 40% in people under 65. Black and ethnic minorities comprise 35% of the population. It is well established in epidemiological data that the risk of CHD is high in Asians and that of stroke is high in Afro-Caribbeans (Balarajan and Raleigh, 1993). The District:
>
> Translates its literature into Asian languages
> GPs are advised by the Family Health Services Authority (FHSA) to carry out opportunistic blood pressure checks on Black and minority ethnic patients
> A healthy eating booklet is produced which includes examples and photos of Asian and Caribbean foods
>
> Is the District meeting the needs of ethnic minority groups? Or is it assuming that because epidemiology identifies Asians and Afro-Caribbeans as a high risk group for CHD and stroke, all ethnic minorities are "in need" of a CHD prevention programme and their needs are the same?

3. To target risk groups

The concept of risk groups has emerged as a means of directing health promotion activities to people who are most in need. Normative needs derived from epidemiological research, which identifies groups with poorer than average health, are often used to establish target groups. For example, lower socio-economic groups at most risk from ill health and premature death are a commonly identified risk group. Comparative need is used to identify at risk groups who have low take-up rates of services. For example, travellers face specific difficulties accessing primary health care services and may, therefore, be a target group. A life cycle approach which identifies the health risks associated with different age groups has also been developed (Pickin and St Leger, 1993).

However, a focus on high-risk groups can lead to "victim-blaming". Health problems are seen as specific to particular groups who may also be seen as responsible through their behaviour for their own ill health. The example of HIV prevention illustrates this problem: gay men and injecting drug users have been the subject of targeted health promotion campaigns. Yet it is not being gay which is a risk but certain sexual activities. Health is frequently seen as a problem for individuals rather than a population issue, hence the emphasis on reducing risk factors. The World Health Organisation advocate a population, rather than a high-risk approach, to promoting health which attempts to alter the lifestyle and environments giving rise to ill health and disease. Many health promoters also reject the notion of targeting because they prefer to work in partnership with groups and communities on the issues *they* define as important.

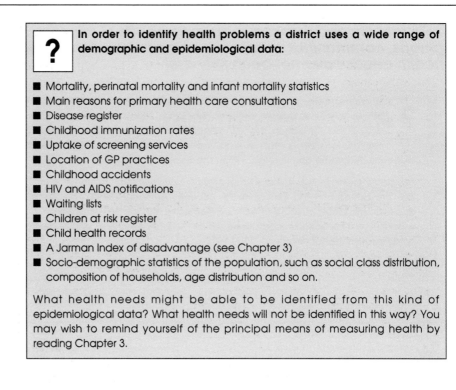

In order to identify health problems a district uses a wide range of demographic and epidemiological data:

- Mortality, perinatal mortality and infant mortality statistics
- Main reasons for primary health care consultations
- Disease register
- Childhood immunization rates
- Uptake of screening services
- Location of GP practices
- Childhood accidents
- HIV and AIDS notifications
- Waiting lists
- Children at risk register
- Child health records
- A Jarman Index of disadvantage (see Chapter 3)
- Socio-demographic statistics of the population, such as social class distribution, composition of households, age distribution and so on.

What health needs might be able to be identified from this kind of epidemiological data? What health needs will not be identified in this way? You may wish to remind yourself of the principal means of measuring health by reading Chapter 3.

4. Resource allocation

The NHS was predicated on the notion that there was an untreated pool of sickness that once treated by a national health service, would diminish. Experience shows that there can be unlimited demand for health care. As health care is provided, so expectations rise; as technology improves people with disabilities and chronic diseases live longer and demand more health care. General improvements in health and living conditions have led to people living longer and an increase in the percentage of older people in the population. It will not be possible to meet all these needs as resources are limited.

Most doctors and health care workers accept that some kind of priority setting or rationing of health care is inevitable. There have always been waiting lists but rationing is a more far-reaching concept. It entails decisions about how much money should be put into different forms of care or treatment. Not only does this raise issues about justice and equity, it also poses the huge dilemma about who decides the priorities for investment. Public views may be very different from those of doctors. For example, infertility treatment may have a high value to individuals but not to society as a whole. Breast screening may be rated highly by the public but not by doctors who are more in a position to question its effectiveness.

In Oregon in the USA a health commission of health care workers and the public devised a complex formula to prioritize health services and decided there were certain services they would not provide. In the UK health care may no longer be free and available to all who need it. Health authorities are beginning to consider particular services which will not be provided as part of the NHS. Cosmetic surgery, for example, may no longer be provided except in exceptional circumstances such as when required as a result of burns or trauma (British Medical Journal, 1993).

? **Consider why limited resources might be more likely to go to a special care baby unit rather than day care for elderly mentally ill people.**

Care for older people is often seen as a low priority because older people are not economically productive and the care may not increase their life expectancy. Those who make rationing decisions will take into account many other factors and your answer will probably include some of the following:

- Costs – the relative costs of different services, and the "opportunity costs" (i.e. if the money is spent on this, what is it not being spent on)
- Numbers – how many people will benefit from the service and will it provide the greatest good for the greatest number
- Effectiveness – what are the likely outcomes of providing care or treatment? Will it promote health, prevent ill health, improve or cure ill health?
- Quality – what areas of health-related quality of life (physical, mental, social, well-being, perception of pain, self-care) will be most affected by the service?

? **How do you account for the low priority accorded to health promotion in terms of NHS funding?**

When we consider the criteria for rationing of health care, we can see why health promotion is a low priority in the NHS – its "Cinderella" service – despite its low costs:

- Health promotion lacks sufficient evidence of its effectiveness
- In the NHS clout is held by doctors not community health care workers
- Health promotion does not have the public appeal of medicine.

The process of assessing need

Individual needs

For those health promoters who work with individual clients, there is increasing recognition of the importance of client participation in the assessment of needs. Nursing practice, for example, has frequently been criticized for being too inflexible and routine – doing things **to** people rather than **with** them. Prescription has now given way to negotiation alongside the move from sick nursing to health nursing. Understanding the thoughts, feelings and experiences of individuals has become an important part of the therapeutic and nursing process.

Research on patient communication has in the past focused on

For what reasons might a client find it difficult to express their needs in a clinical situation?

why **patients** do not comply with medical advice (Ley,1988) but the emphasis is shifting and increasingly health care workers are receiving training in communication skills. This kind of training teaches the health care worker how to put clients at their ease, and how to ask open-ended questions which elicit clients' views and perceptions about their health and health behaviour. Many health promoters with individual clients can benefit from counselling techniques which use non-directive questions and emphasize listening skills.

What health care workers often find when they carry out a needs assessment with a client is that their perception differs from that of the client. Clients' need for information is often underestimated and in health care settings, this may mean information is confined to ward or clinic routines. Health care workers value information in so far as it increases compliance. In a study of women's information needs regarding the menopause, it was found that women wanted far greater detail particularly concerning hormone replacement therapy which would allow them to make a more informed choice (Farrant and Russell,1985). The dictate that health education publications should be short and simple, although widespread, has little basis in research that has looked at information needs from a target audience perspective. Instead, it can be seen as reflecting, in part at least, "broader ideological perspectives of the professional middle classes and being largely perpetuated, within health education, by methodological misconceptions – particularly concerning the nature, function and applicability of readability tests" (Farrant and Russell, 1985).

Despite the greater emphasis on being client-centred in all health, welfare and education work, health promoters tend to assess needs in relation to the service they provide. Very often client needs are seen as information because it is possible to provide this whereas the satisfaction of physical needs (as in Maslow's hierarchy) may seem beyond their scope.

> **?** A pilot project aims to help patients to decide their own clinical treatment where genuine choices are available. Patients with borderline blood pressure problems key in their individual information to an interactive video which then recommends which of the three available choices is most suitable. The choices are: to watch and wait; to change their lifestyle through diet and exercise; or to go on to medication.
>
> What might be the advantages and disadvantages of this method of individual needs assessment?

Public views

The NHS reforms of the 1990s place an emphasis on the need to involve local people in all stages of the commissioning process. For many health authorities this is part of a formal exercise conducted in a top-down way. Frequently the consultation is confined to issues relating to patient satisfaction with services and particularly the hotel aspects of care.

There is, however, a commitment on paper to achieving as wide a range of views as possible. For example, the Health of the Nation strategy handbook on mental health cites the following organizations to consider during consultation:

Patient councils and advocates
National and local voluntary sector, e.g. MIND, CRUSE, Samaritans
Community health councils
Carers' groups.

However, the process of consultation often views people as the passive providers of information and not as active participants in the process. Levenson and Joule (1992) identify four models of user involvement in NHS planning:

"Tell me you love me" in which a survey is drawn up by NHS managers on patient satisfaction
"Kill them with kindness" in which the public are invited indiscriminately to all planning meetings but rarely encouraged to be fully involved
"The Godfather" in which a community leader is identified and this person becomes the conduit to black and minority ethnic groups
"Puppet Show" in which a group is identified as giving the views of the community.

Health and local authorities are beginning to use a range of initiatives to achieve a wider voice rather than one-off consultation exercises.

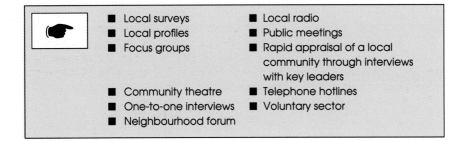

■ Local surveys
■ Local profiles
■ Focus groups

■ Local radio
■ Public meetings
■ Rapid appraisal of a local community through interviews with key leaders

■ Community theatre
■ One-to-one interviews
■ Neighbourhood forum

■ Telephone hotlines
■ Voluntary sector

It is important that this is a process of participation and a sharing of information which means that health authorities act on the information received, and identify where early changes can be made and where areas are beyond their control.

A locality management group of a GP forum held a focus group discussion on womens' knowledge of the contraceptive pill as part of a series of focus groups in its effort to improve client involvement in the assessment of health needs. The issues raised by the focus group have formed the basis for a questionnaire which is being given to women who present to their GP or family planning clinic for a repeat prescription of the contraceptive pill.

 A self-completion questionnaire with two reminders was sent to a random 30 000 residents in South East Thames Regional Health Authority. It included sections on health status, service use, accidents, smoking, alcohol consumption and some socio-demographic characteristics.

 In Mid-Essex the community has been involved in setting health care priorities through:

- Workshop meetings
- Questionnaires
- Small group discussions with the community health council
- Discussions with voluntary groups
- Discussion with GPs
- Rapid appraisal of localities
- Informing the community by making the Public Health Report more accessible.

Professional views

In the drafting of health plans to meet community needs, it is important to include the views and experience of health promoters who work in primary health care, in schools, in environmental health, in housing, or on the streets as youth workers, community workers or police officers. Until such time as sharing information and Healthy Alliances are a matter of course, this expertise can be lost. The standardization of information-gathering by different agencies will also aid intelligence on community needs.

Whose needs count?

Moves to participation either in community affairs or health care cannot involve everyone. There will be individuals and groups who are not able to take advantage of opportunities for expression. These are the potential and future users of a service; those who are not part of an established group; those who are not deemed sufficiently "rational" to have a view such as children, people with learning difficulties and sometimes older people. Participation obviously favours those with the most influence and loudest voices.

One health authority undertook a rapid appraisal exercise to ascertain its community's perceptions of priority needs and the strength of feeling around these areas. The key informants were deemed to be:

- Those who had some professional knowledge, e.g. social workers
- Leaders within the community, e.g. those who run self-help groups
- People centrally placed in their work, e.g. shopkeepers.

Popay and Williams (1992) describe examples of popular epidemiology where a community gets a health issue acknowledged by compiling evidence to substantiate their views. They term this a "competing rationality". For example, people in Camelford in Cornwall documented the symptoms they experienced when 20 tonnes of aluminium sulphate was accidentally tipped into the water tank supplying their homes.

Setting priorities

Since the publication of a national health strategy in *The Health of the Nation*, many health promoters will find that they are working to the five target areas identified in that document. The criteria used for setting these priorities were:

1. The area should be a major cause of premature death or avoidable ill health in the population as a whole or amongst specific groups of people
2. Effective interventions should be possible offering scope for improvements in health
3. It should be possible to set objectives and targets in the area and monitor progress towards achievement through indicators.

In addition there may be locally determined priorities of specific health issues such as diabetes or particular population groups such as older people.

However, in most people's work a whole range of other criteria may influence the setting of priorities.

? **A health promotion manager working with a small team is deciding the annual plan. The health authority has adopted all the Health of the Nation targets and identified the prevention of coronary heart disease and stroke as a main priority. The area is a seaside town with a stable population. It has a high proportion of older people and low income Department of Social Security accommodation. There is a newly appointed HIV prevention coordinator whose post is funded for 2 years from monies ring-fenced for HIV and AIDS. Through the health promotion inter-disciplinary forum, the community nurse manager has identified that many older people are drinking heavily. There have been three child drownings so far this year. The Health Education Authority has**

> **(cont.)**
>
> **informed you that in December it is World AIDS Day, in March it is National No Smoking Day, in June it is Drinkwise Day, in November it is European Drug Prevention Week, and in addition it is European Year for Health and Safety.**
>
> How will the manager decide between these competing priorities?
>
> - A national primary target of reducing CHD in those under 65 by 10%
> - A national theme
> - A major determinant of health in the area, i.e. age and poverty
> - Pragmatism on the basis of available skills and interests
> - Cost
> - Longer term strategy
> - Cost-effectiveness and what is amenable to change and evaluation
> - Client choice
> - Professional's views.

Conclusion

- **What reasons can you think of to explain why these groups are hard to reach?**
- **Can you think of any other groups that might be hard to reach?**

The process of encouraging consumerism and participation in public services by identifying and understanding individual and community needs has led to attempts to make such services more flexible. So we find as part of the nursing process clients being encouraged to identify aspects of their situation that they deem harmful to their health. We find health authorities using a variety of methods to ascertain the views, beliefs and health behaviours of their population in addition to the objective measures yielded by epidemiology. We find voluntary and community groups being required as part of their funding to monitor not only their clients' use of the service but also their health needs.

These moves are to be applauded but there are two major problems that arise in this process of needs assessment. Firstly, are the views which are heard representative? It is very difficult to get a cross-section of a community and there are some groups of people who are hard to reach. These include homeless people, unemployed people, and people from Black and ethnic minority groups.

Some groups comprise individuals who may have a similar experience of health services because of a defining characteristic of being unemployed or homeless, but they do not have a collective voice or access to their views. Other groups may be informal with no recognized meeting place. Many groups may be wary of formal and statutory bodies.

Secondly, the public sector, but particularly the NHS, works within a scientific, objective framework for planning which makes it hard to incorporate the subjective experiences of people.

The challenge for health promotion is to define needs assessment in its own terms. In particular when population or community needs are assessed, we should look at felt needs as well as epidemiology. When needs are translated into action, we should complement and augment a medical approach with intersectoral planning to ensure maximum participation.

Questions for further discussion

■ How useful is the concept of need as a basis for planning health promotion interventions?
■ How would you go about assessing the needs of:
  ■ Women who inject drugs?
  ■ Young asthmatics?
  ■ Carers of older people?

Summary

This chapter has discussed the ways in which need is defined. We have seen that perceptions of need vary according to whether these are client or professional views, and how the assessment is made – clients' expressed views; levels of service use; epidemiological and social data. The chapter concludes that need is relative, and influenced by values and attitudes as well as the historical context. It also considers the relevance of health promotion to meeting certain needs.

Further reading

Bradshaw J (1972) "The concept of social need", *New Society*, **19**, 640–643.

This attempt to define need is widely used and although it lacks a theoretical base, it recognizes that "need" involves value judgements by health and social care workers.

Buchan H (1990) "Needs assessment made simple", *Health Services Journal,* February 15.

The first of a series of six articles which explore ways in which

NHS purchasers can assess the health needs of the district.

Butler JR (1987) *An Apple a Day? A Study of Lifestyles and Health in Canterbury and Thanet,* University of Kent/Canterbury and Thanet Health Authority.

Liddiard P (1988) *Milton Keynes Felt Needs Project,* Department of Health and Social Welfare, Open University.

Two examples of health needs assessment using survey and qualitative methods.

McIver S (1991) *Obtaining the Views of Users of Health*

Services, London, King's Fund.

NHS Management Executive (1992) *Local Voices: Involving the Local Community in Purchasing Decisions*, NHS Management Executive.

Advice for NHS managers on ways to increase community participation in decisions regarding health care provision.

References

Acheson D (1982) Public Health in England, *Report of the Committee of Inquiry into the Future*

Development of the Public Health Function, London, HMSO.

Armstrong P (1982) "The myth of meeting needs in adult education and community development", *Critical Social Policy*, **2** (2), 24–37.

Balarajan R and Raleigh VS (1993) *Ethnicity and Health*, London, Department of Health.

Bradshaw J (1972) "The concept of social need", *New Society*, **19**, 640–643.

British Medical Association (1993) *Rationing in Action*, London, BMJ Publishing.

Department of Health (1989) *Working for Patients*, London, HMSO.

Farrant W and Russell J (1985) *HEC Publications: A Case Study in the Production, Distribution and Use of Health Information*, London, HEC.

Illich I, Zola IK, McKnight J, Caplan J and Shaiken H (1977) *Disabling Professions*, London, Boyars.

Levenson R and Joule N (1992) *Listening to People: User Involvement in the NHS*, London, Greater London Association of Community Health Councils.

Ley P (1988) *Communicating with Patients – Improving Communication, Satisfaction and Compliance*, London, Croom Helm.

Maslow AH (1954) *Motivation and Personality*, New York, Harper & Row.

NHS Management Executive (1992) *Local Voices: Involving the Local Community in Purchasing Decisions*, Leeds, NHS Management Executive.

Oliver (1993) *Psychology and Health Care.*

Pickin C and St Leger S (1993) *Assessing Health Need Using the Life Cycle Framework*, Milton Keynes, Open University Press.

Popay J and Williams G (1992) "Involving local people in health gain: the contribution of lay epidemiology", *Health For All 2000 News*, **19**.

Tannahill A (1992) "Epidemiology and health promotion", in Bunton R and Macdonald G (eds) *Health Promotion: Disciplines and Diversity*, London, Routledge.

Tudor Hart (1971) "The inverse care law", *Lancet*, **i**, 405

World Health Organisation (WHO) (1978) *Report on the Primary Health Care Conference: Alma Ata*, Geneva, World Health Organisation.

Planning health promotion interventions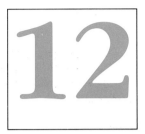

Overview

We have seen in Chapter 11 how needs assessment and targeting may be carried out, and the importance of carrying out this process and being clear about the context in which this is done. This chapter extends this discussion, and follows on from Chapter 11. First, definitions of planning are given and the reasons for planning discussed. After considering the characteristics of planning frameworks, four different planning models are presented, and the advantages and limitations of using each are considered.

Key points
■ Reasons for planning
■ Rational planning models
■ Integrated health promotion planning
■ Planning models:
■ Ewles and Simnett
■ PRECEDE
■ Tones
■ Berry
■ Contract specification
■ Quality

Definitions

Planning is one of those terms which is used in many different ways. Other related terms are used in equally imprecise ways, so that often the same activity is labelled in different ways by different people. There are no hard and fast rules about the way terms are used, but the following definitions are presented as a means of clarifying the differences between related activities. These are the definitions we shall be using in this chapter.

Plan – how to get from your starting point to your end point and what you want to achieve.

Policy – guidelines for practice which set broad goals and the framework for action.

Programme – overall outline of action. The collection of activities in a planned sequence leading to a defined goal or goals.

Strategy – the methods to be used in achieving goals.

Priority – the first claim for consideration.

Aim – broad goal.

Objective – specific goal to be achieved.

> ☞ **Judy has been given a remit to develop a health promotion *programme* with the *aim* of reducing the suicide rate. Her health authority's *policy* includes a commitment to equal opportunities. She decides her *priority* area will be unemployed people, who are known to be at increased risk of suicide. Judy's *objectives* are to: (1) set up a support group for unemployed people; and (2) to provide specialist counselling services. Her *strategy* is to network with existing community groups, and to recruit and train volunteer counsellors.**

Reasons for planning

Health promoters usually have no problem in finding things to do which seem reasonable. Work areas are inherited from others, delegated from more senior members of the workplace or demanded by clients. It is possible to be kept very busy reacting to all these pressures, and planning health promotion interventions may seem a luxury or a waste of time. However, there are sound reasons for planning health promotion or being proactive in your work practice. Planning is important because it helps direct resources to where they will have most impact. Planning ensures that health promotion is not overlooked but is prioritized as a work activity.

Planning takes different forms and is used at different levels. It may be used to provide the best services or care for an individual client, as in the nursing process, or planning may be for group activities, such as antenatal classes. Planning may also refer to large-scale health promotion interventions targeted at whole populations.

Planning models

Rational planning models provide a means to guide choices so that decisions are made which represent the best way to achieve desired results.

> "The 'rational' approach suggests that the whole range of options should be identified and considered before a comprehensive programme is drawn up" (McCarthy, 1982, p.10).

Planning involves several key stages or logical stepping stones which enable the health promoter to achieve a desired result. The benefit is being clear about what it is you want to achieve, i.e. the purpose of any intervention. Planning entails:

1. An assessment of need.
2. Setting aims – what is is you intend to achieve.
3. Setting objectives – precise outcomes. Objectives should be SMART: Specific, Measurable, Achievable, Realistic, Timescale.

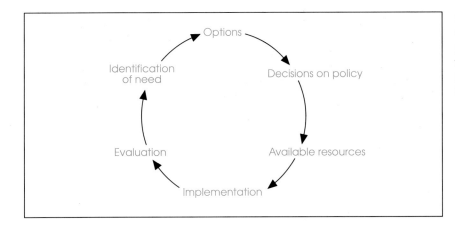

Figure 12.1 McCarthy's model for rational health planning. Reproduced with permission from the King's Fund Centre from McCarthy (1982).

4. Deciding which methods or strategies will achieve your objectives.
5. Evaluating outcomes in order to make improvements in the future.

Some planning models are presented in a linear fashion. Others show a circular process to indicate that any evaluation feeds back into the process (see Figure 12.1).

> **?**   **What do you think would be the best starting point for planning an intervention or programme? Why?**
>
> **Think of any planned activities you have been involved with. What was the starting point? Why?**

However, in real life, planning is often piecemeal or incremental. There is no grand design, but circumstances dictate many small reactive decisions:

> "The 'incremental' approach suggests that planning is necessarily based on limited information, and that the uncertainty of the future makes small decisions preferable to grand plans" (McCarthy, 1982, p.10).

Tannahill (1990) argues that what is needed is an integrated planning framework. Planning for health education is part of the broader task of health promotion and should seek to enhance good communication. Health-oriented health education is to be preferred to the narrower programmes which focus on diseases or risk factors. Tannahill states that disease-oriented or risk-factor-oriented health education tends to be prescriptive in tone and is apt to be duplicated by different professional groups. The public response may be to withdraw from the resulting proliferation of messages which are often inconsistent. He argues that integrated health-oriented health education which focuses on key settings and key groups is the preferred option (Figure 12.2). This needs to be

- Which do you think is preferable, rational or incremental planning?
- Which are the most important factors to consider?

Figure 12.2 Tannahill's
integrated planning
framework (from
Tannahill, 1990).

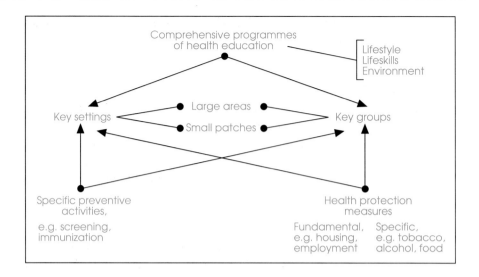

Figure 12.2 Tannahill's integrated planning framework (from Tannahill, 1990).

complemented by preventive and protective health promotion measures.

McCarthy (1982) and Tannahill (1990) argue that planning should be a rational, organized and integrated activity. French and Milner (1993) state that current health promotion practice is incapable of having a major impact on the health status of populations, and that planning to achieve these goals is illusory. In real life planning is often carried out on a smaller scale and is subject to practical constraints. For example, planning in real life often follows the allocation of resources instead of dictating resources. They propose a model of health development which is "a systematic but non-linear planning process" (Figure 12.3) (French and Milner, 1993, p.100). Health development focuses on health or well-being at the level of individuals or small groups. It is broader than health education but not as all-embracing as health promotion. French and Milner claim that using the health development model will enable a more flexible and collaborative work practice to emerge.

Other models seek to provide more detailed guidance on the stages involved in planning health promotion interventions. We shall examine four of the best known models: Ewles and Simnett,

Figure 12.3 French and Milner's real planning model (from French and Milner, 1993).

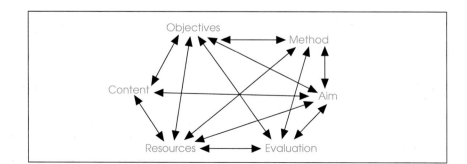

PRECEDE, Tones and Berry. The advantages and limitations of each model will be considered.

Ewles and Simnett

Ewles and Simnett (1992) provide a straightforward and popular model, which is reproduced in Figure 12.4.

The first stage is needs assessment and the identification of priorities, which was considered in the previous chapter. This needs assessment will identify certain goals or aims for health promotion. To be of use in planning, these aims need to be made more specific, or translated into objectives.

Setting objectives is a key stage in planning. Objectives are the specific goals to be achieved, and the measurement of the extent to which this happens is evaluation. There is a balance to be struck between setting objectives which are realistic but also challenging.

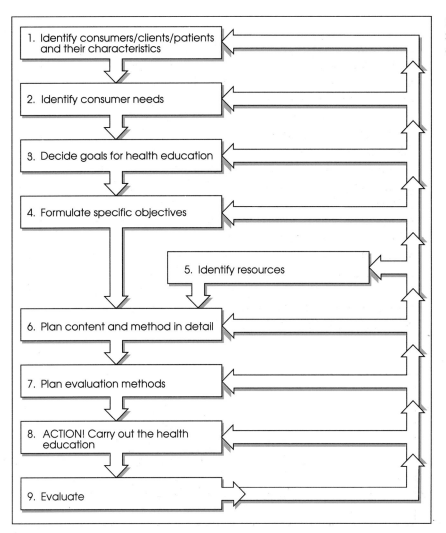

Figure 12.4 Ewles and Simnett planning model (from Ewles and Simnett, 1992).

Objectives state what outcomes should result from an intervention. Educational objectives should be relevant, realizable and measurable. Ewles and Simnett (1992) identify three types of educational objectives:

1. Cognitive objectives concerning increased levels of knowledge
2. Affective objectives concerning attitudes and beliefs
3. Skills or psycho-motor objectives concerning skills acquisition and competence.

Health promotion objectives may in addition include:

4. Behaviour change including changes in lifestyles and increased take-up of services
5. Policy objectives concerning changes in policy
6. Process objectives concerning increases in participation and working together
7. Environmental objectives concerning changing the environment to make it more healthy.

? **The following are objectives set for a health promotion programme to increase people's exercise levels. Which objectives are specific, realistic and measurable?**

■ To increase the amount of regular exercise taken
■ To facilitate a more positive attitude towards exercise on the part of young women
■ To increase young people's knowledge of the effects of exercise
■ To increase the facilities available for exercise in the community
■ To reduce mortality from CHD
■ To establish a local multi-agency health and exercise group
■ To increase take up of exercise facilities.

The first objective is too vague whilst the fifth is unrealistic. The other objectives are more appropriate but would require different methods and timescales.

The next stage is to decide which methods to use. This choice will be decided in part by external considerations, such as the amount of funding, or the particular expertise of the health promoter. However, the type of methods chosen should also reflect the objectives set. Certain methods go with certain objectives but would be quite inappropriate for other objectives. For example, participative small group work is effective at changing attitudes but a more formal teaching session would be more effective if specific knowledge is to be imparted. Community development is effective at increasing community involvement and participation but would not be appropriate if local government policy change is the objective. The mass media is effective in raising people's awareness of health issues but ineffective in persuading people to change their behaviour. So the next stage in planning is deciding which methods would be the logical choice given your objectives. You may then find you have to compromise owing to constraints of time, resources or skills, but this compromise should concern the amount of input, or the use of complementary methods. It should not mean that you end up using inappropriate methods which are unlikely to achieve your objectives.

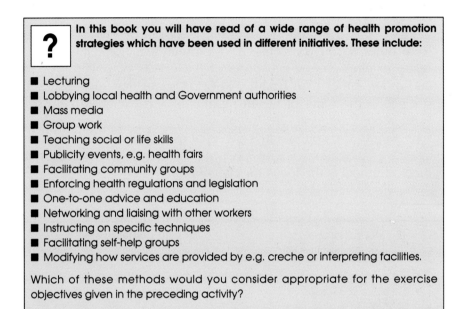

? In this book you will have read of a wide range of health promotion strategies which have been used in different initiatives. These include:

- Lecturing
- Lobbying local health and Government authorities
- Mass media
- Group work
- Teaching social or life skills
- Publicity events, e.g. health fairs
- Facilitating community groups
- Enforcing health regulations and legislation
- One-to-one advice and education
- Networking and liaising with other workers
- Instructing on specific techniques
- Facilitating self-help groups
- Modifying how services are provided by e.g. creche or interpreting facilities.

Which of these methods would you consider appropriate for the exercise objectives given in the preceding activity?

When objectives and methods have been decided the next stage is to consider whether any specific resources are needed to implement the strategy. Resources include funding, people's skills and expertise, and materials such as leaflets and learning packs.

Once you have decided on your target group, objectives, methods and resources, the type of intervention required should be apparent. You will need to plan a timetable to show what needs to be done when. You may also identify interim indicators of progress to show if you are proceeding as planned. The question of evaluation will need to be considered. This issue is discussed in detail in the following chapter.

The Ewles and Simnett model is very practical and flexible. It is a useful guide which, with minor modifications, may be used for a wide variety of interventions ranging from the small-scale planning of one to one sessions to large scale campaigns.

PRECEDE

PRECEDE stands for Predisposing Reinforcing and Enabling Causes in Educational Diagnosis and Evaluation. This model was developed by Green *et al.* (1980) and has been used extensively in health education interventions. Figure 12.5 gives a diagrammatic representation of PRECEDE.

Phase 1 is the identification of a population's concerns and problems relating to their quality of life. The starting point is a community's subjective perceptions, which may be determined in several ways. Chapter 11 considers a range of methods to identify community health needs.

Phase 2 is the identification and isolation of health problems from other social problems. A community's major concerns may relate to employment prospects or the effects of poverty, or law and order, rather than health. PRECEDE states that such issues are not within the remit of health promotion and excludes them from further consideration. Health problems are defined not only by reference to the community's perceptions, but also by reference to available epidemiological or medical data. Health as defined by the medical model is the focus for intervention.

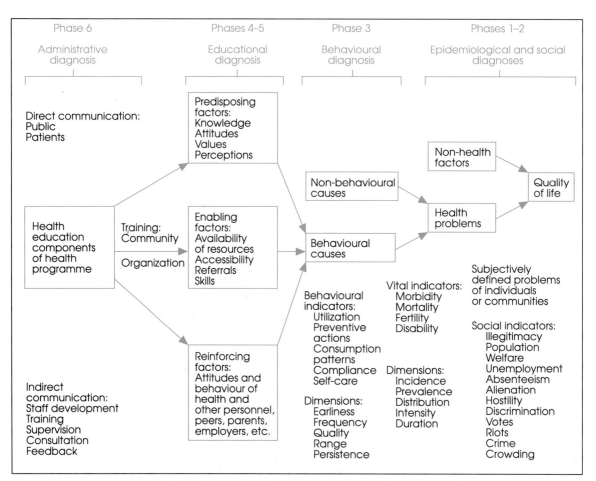

Figure 12.5 PRECEDE planning model (from Green *et al.*, 1980).

Phase 3 is the behavioural diagnosis. Non-behavioural causes of health problems, such as unhealthy environments or policies, are excluded at this stage. Behavioural causes need to be carefully identified and ranked in order to progress to phase 4, which is the identification of three categories of factors which affect behaviour. Predisposing factors are a person's beliefs, values and attitudes which will affect their motivation to change. Enabling factors refer to the skills and resources which are necessary to allow the enactment of motivated behaviour. Social factors, such as income or accessibility of services are resources enabling the achievement of desired behaviour change. Personal factors, such as an adequate level of knowledge and skills are also enabling factors. Enabling factors, if absent, will be "barriers" which need to be overcome in order to enable behaviour change to occur. Reinforcing factors refer to the feedback received from significant others, which may help or hinder the process of behaviour change.

Phase 4 is the analysis of these three categories of factors and the selection of the most important factors. Phase 5 follows automatically and is the decision of which factors are to be the focus of the intervention. The type and extent of resources available will help inform this decision. Phase 6 again follows logically from the previous phases, and is the development and implementation of an appropriate educational intervention. The management and administration of the intervention is also considered at this stage. Administrative diagnosis includes assessment of resources and organizational relationships, and the production of a timetable. Phase 7 is the evaluation of the intervention, although Green *et al.* (1980) stress that this should be an integrated activity addressed throughout the planning process.

The intention is that using PRECEDE will guide the health educator to the most effective type of intervention. Using knowledge drawn from epidemiology, social psychology, education and management studies, the health educator can arrive at an optimum intervention. The model is said to be based on a complementary mix of expertise drawn from these different disciplines. Green *et al.* (1980, p.11) claim that PRECEDE "has served as a successful model in a number of rigorously evaluated 'real world' clinical trials".

In practice, the model is often modified and is rarely used as illustrated. For example, it is unusual to begin the process of planning with as open an agenda as "quality of life". Priority topics, target groups or settings have more often been identified at the outset. For example, the "Health of the Nation" targets (Department of Health, 1992) (see page 51) have stimulated a range of planned health promotion activities. These activities are in response to selected objectives concerning preventable diseases which have been defined by professionals. So in practice PRECEDE often begins at the behavioural diagnosis rather than the needs assessment phase.

PRECEDE as a health education planning model mirrors the medical world. The planning process is dominated by experts. The general public may be involved in identifying problems, but the ways and means of tackling these problems are to be determined by experts. The focus is on achieving behavioural change at the level of individuals or groups. The social, political and environmental context of health is systematically screened out by the model in phases one and two. To some extent this may be explained by PRECEDE being a health education rather than a health promotion planning model. A model developed specifically for health education cannot be expected to apply to other forms of health promotion but, for most people, education, even if it does not include changing the environment, does include clarifying values, beliefs and attitudes, facilitating self-empowerment and supporting autonomy. In PRECEDE these activities tend to be subordinated to the primary aim of behaviour change. It could be argued that PRECEDE is a model dominated by social psychology and behavioural perspectives rather than educational perspectives, and that the label is therefore misleading. PRECEDE is, however, a highly structured planning model which ensures that certain issues are considered. If the objective is behaviour change, then PRECEDE is a useful model to follow.

Tones

Tones (1974, revised in Steel, 1986) provides a planning model for health education which is illustrated in Figure 12.6.

The first stage in Tones' model is not an assessment of needs but the identification of goals. Four categories of goals are given: medically defined problems, medically defined problem behaviour, lay-defined problems, and positive health states. Goals are not defined solely in terms of problems and positive health is included as a potential goal.

The next stage is to translate these goals into educational aims. These aims are further refined into objectives by considering the special characteristics of the target group. In Chapter 10 the ways in which people can be helped to change was explored with reference to models of behaviour change. The Health Action Model highlighted the role of group norms and lay referral systems in this process. "Health career" refers to how someone constructs and negotiates the story and meaning of their health by reference to significant events, such as contacts with health workers. Objectives need to be negotiated with, and be meaningful for, the target group. Objectives are pretested with the target population in order to ensure their acceptability and appropriateness.

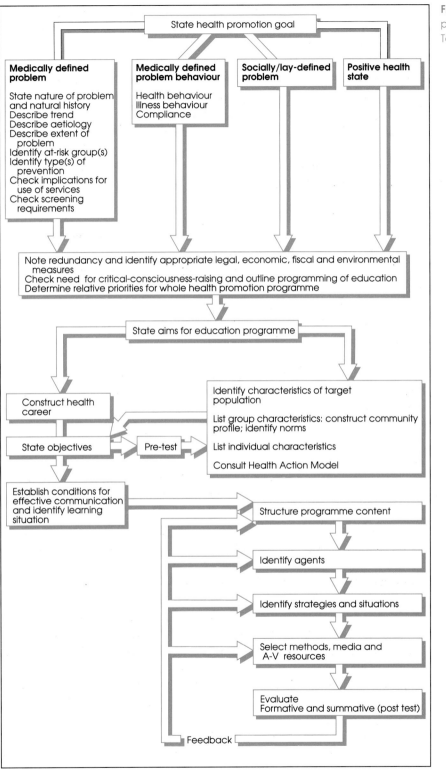

Figure 12.6 Tones' planning model (from Tones, 1974).

The next phase is to structure the programme content in the light of educational theory. This leads on to the identification of agents, the identification of strategies and situations, and the selection of appropriate methods, media and audio-visual resources. Evaluation is the last stage of the process, but feedback from evaluation should then inform the programme content and design.

Tones' model is again primarily educational, and shares some characteristics with Ewles and Simnett's model. It differs in being more complicated to follow and in starting out with health promotion goals rather than needs assessment. This has the effect of making the model more expert-oriented or top-down. Lay-defined problems are one source of health promotion goals but the process as a whole is controlled by the health promoter. Community characteristics are identified because they will enable more appropriate objectives to be set not because the process of consultation is seen as valuable in its own right. Tones' model also shares similarities with PRECEDE, in particular the systematic screening out of non-educational types of health promotion intervention. The major difference is that Tones' model focuses on education rather than behaviour change.

Berry

Berry's model (1986) provides a framework for district health authorities to use when planning health promotion and preventive medicine programmes. Figure 12.7 is a diagrammatic representation of Berry's model.

The first stage is the setting up of working groups that then go on to review the problem, using epidemiological and research data. This is followed by the identification of the project. Project objectives need to be identified, and should refer to changes in knowledge, attitudes, behaviour or health status. Target groups and estimated costs also need specifying at this stage. Stages 5 and 6 focus on identifying an appropriate evaluation strategy, estimating costs and carrying out baseline studies to provide the control data. Stage 7 is the design of intervention material which needs to be pretested or piloted with the target group to assess its effectiveness. Material may need to be modified in the light of this pretesting.

Stage 9 is the actual implementation of the project. This is followed by monitoring the changes which have occurred and an estimation of the costs of achieving such change. This information is used to compile an evaluation report which in turn contributes to the working group reviewing the project policy and deciding whether it should be repeated, and whether any modifications are necessary. The final stage is the overall review of the project in the light of its objectives and overall policy.

Berry's model is grounded in the organizational context and is

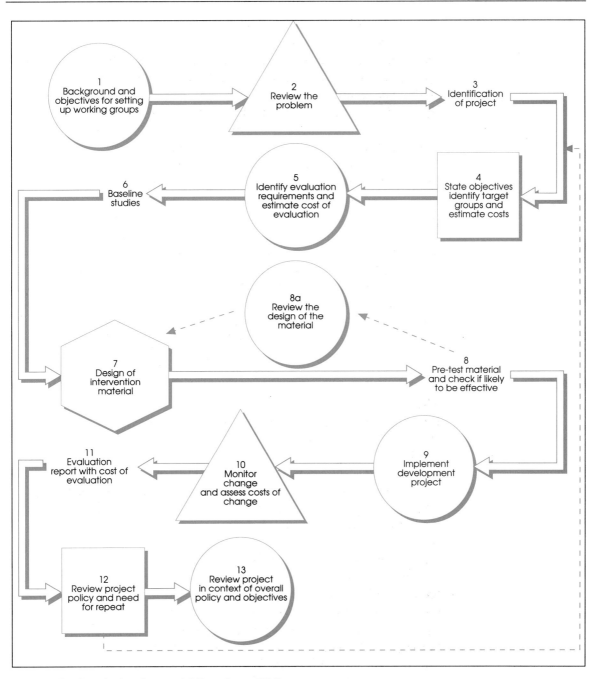

Figure 12.7 Berry's planning model (from Berry, 1986).

applicable to health promotion interventions as well as health education interventions. The emphasis on costings and the need for rigour in setting objectives and identifying change arise in part from this organizational context. Management aspects of the planning process are highlighted. For example, starting with the setting up of working groups is a managerial solution to the problem of health promotion being interdisciplinary in nature.

Berry's model is another example of a top-down, expert-oriented planning framework. Problems are to be determined by experts and there is no real community consultation, only the piloting of intervention materials. Its strength is that it could lead to a higher profile for health promotion, if it becomes an integrated part of the services provided by an organization.

Putting health promotion into contracts

We have looked at ways of planning health promotion interventions in a rational way. In practice, health promotion must establish its role within the NHS. One way of planning for health promotion is by putting it into contracts. The recent NHS reforms have led to a purchaser/provider split, whereby purchasing health authorities establish contracts with provider authorities to provide specified services for their populations. The "Health of the Nation" strategy and targets provide a rationale and impetus for putting health promotion into contracts. Killoran (1991) suggests that there are three approaches to tapping health promotion into contracts.

1. All contracts can refer to health promotion by, for example, ensuring that service delivery takes account of factors, such as a health-promoting environment, patient education and equal access. This is often included as part of the quality specifications which apply to all contracts. Quality has been defined as:

> ". . . the totality of the features and characteristics of a product or service that bear on its ability to satisfy stated or implied need" (British Standards Institute, 1978).

The core principles of quality have been defined as (Evans *et al.* 1994):

■ Equity – that users have equal access and/or equal benefit from services
■ Effectiveness – that services achieve their intended objectives
■ Efficiency – that services achieve maximum benefit for minimum cost
■ Accessibility – that a service is easily available to users in terms of time, distance and ethos
■ Appropriatenesss – that a service is that which the users require
■ Acceptability – that services satisfy the reasonable expectations of users
■ Responsiveness – that services adapt to the expressed needs of users.

> **?** Compare the list above with the WHO criteria for health promotion on pages 74–75. What do you notice?

Quality expresses a notion of "fit for the purpose" but also conveys a notion of excellence. Applying the notion of quality to work practice is difficult. One means of trying to do this is through quality assurance which has been defined as:

> "a systematic process through which achievable and desirable levels of quality are described, the extent to which these levels are achieved is assessed, and action taken following assessment to enable them to be realized" (Wright and Whittington, 1992).

Quality assurance is an ongoing process of continual assessment and improvement of practice. Figure 12.8 gives a diagrammatic representation of the quality assurance cycle.

Standards are agreed levels of performance within available resources. Criteria specify the precise levels of performance to be achieved in order to meet standards. Criteria may refer to necessary

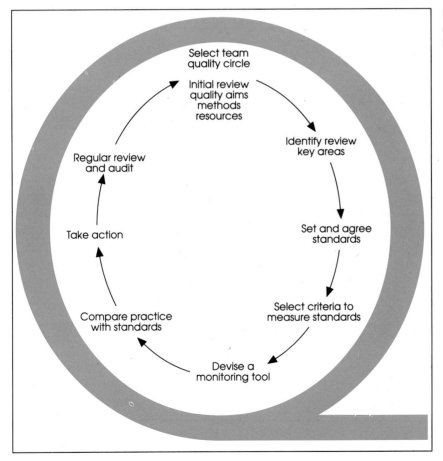

Figure 12.8 The quality assurance cycle (from Boyd, 1994).

resources, how the process is to be carried out or expected outcomes.

2. Contracts can also specify certain activities to be undertaken in support of the major "Health of the Nation" targets. The following example states the purchasing intentions of one health authority with reference to the "Health of the Nation" target to reduce mortality from CHD.

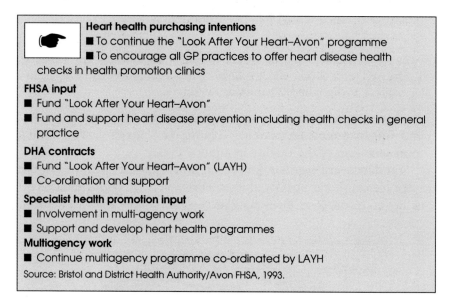

Heart health purchasing intentions
- To continue the "Look After Your Heart–Avon" programme
- To encourage all GP practices to offer heart disease health checks in health promotion clinics

FHSA input
- Fund "Look After Your Heart–Avon"
- Fund and support heart disease prevention including health checks in general practice

DHA contracts
- Fund "Look After Your Heart–Avon" (LAYH)
- Co-ordination and support

Specialist health promotion input
- Involvement in multi-agency work
- Support and develop heart health programmes

Multiagency work
- Continue multiagency programme co-ordinated by LAYH

Source: Bristol and District Health Authority/Avon FHSA, 1993.

3. Contracts may include guidelines for the development of health promotion services, e.g. the establishment of specialist support services incorporating training and resources.

Once contracts have been specified and agreed, ongoing monitoring takes place to ensure contracts are being met. A range of indicators may be used to see whether planned targets for activity are being met. Activities may refer to prevention policies and the delivery of services including education, screening, treatment and rehabilitation. An example is shown in Table 12.1.

Table 12.1 Monitoring of the CHD programme: West Dorset Health Authority (from Killoran, 1992).

Prevention
- Annual positive health analysis of knowledge, attitudes, and behaviour from survey and general practice data.
- Annual reports of action and outcomes from PATCH teams.
- Number of organizations employing over 750 employees that have signed the LAYH Charter with effective monitoring of key activities.
- Details of health promotion marketing and feedback analysis.

Education and health marketing
- Personal requests to health promotion service for information.
- Parent views of new Parentcraft package.
- Detail of identified target markets, analysis of consumer views on the marketing.

Investigations
- Annual laboratory report on cholesterol screening.
- FHSA monitoring of cholesterol screening referrals.
- Referrals for exercise ECG – exception reporting for delayed investigation.
- Waiting times for angiography.

Treatment
- Percentage of coronary patient admissions treated with streptokinase/alternative drug.
- Waiting time for coronary artery bypass surgery operations.
- Number of coronary artery bypass operations for West Dorset residents each year.

Rehabilitation
- Percentage uptake of exercise clinic programme.
- Patient comments on CHD guide to daily living.

Overall monitoring
- Number of deaths by age and sex, standardized mortality ratios.
- Number of admissions and admission rates of patients with a diagnosis of acute myocardial infarction and of unstable angina by age and sex.
- Number of new cases and incidence rates by age and sex of angina from selected practices and acute myocardial infarction with appropriate record systems.
- Positive health survey data monitoring for each PATCH.

Review and audit are more infrequent and systematic appraisals of practice. The idea of peer audit is becoming more popular in health promotion, and the Society of Health Education/Promotion Specialists (SHEPS) has developed an audit scheme.

Conclusion

There are sound reasons for adopting a rational planning model to structure health promotion interventions. However, no one model is right for all circumstances. The Ewles and Simnett model is a good all purpose framework, whilst Tones' model is specifically adapted for educational interventions. PRECEDE is more geared towards behaviour change, and Berry's model is more appropriate for planning within the context of a large organization.

In reality, planning health promotion is a more complex process than the planning models suggest. This is because rational decision-making is only one factor in determining what happens. Many other factors are also important, including historical precedent, enthusiasms of key people and the political context. So it is unlikely that any health promotion intervention proceeds exactly along the lines indicated by a planning model, but this does not mean models are not useful. Models help structure activities and can act as a checklist to ensure important stages are not missed out. They are there to be modified in the light of experience, not to act as strait-jackets.

The "Health of the Nation" targets and strategy provides, for the first time, a priority and impetus for developing health promotion nationwide. Contract specification in the new NHS structure provides an important means of tapping health promotion into the purchasing and provision of health services. Chapter 14 goes on to discuss the evaluation stage. Evaluating interventions, and being able to determine to what extent health promotion is successful in achieving its objectives, is the key to establishing health promotion as a central plank of health work.

Question for further discussion

■ What factors would you take into account when planning a health promotion intervention?

Summary

This chapter has clarified the terminology used in the planning process and discussed the reasons for planning health promotion interventions. Four planning models which have been developed specifically for health promotion have been discussed in greater detail. The use of contract specifications to tap health promotion into the planning cycles of large organizations such as the NHS has been reviewed.

Further reading

Berry J (1986) "Project health: a step-by-step planning guide for health promotion and preventive medicine programmes", *Health Education Journal*, **45**, 109–111.

This provides a more detailed account of Berry's model.

Evans D, Head M and Speller V (1994) *Assuring Quality in Health Promotion*, Wessex Institute of Public Health Medicine/Health Education Authority.

A comprehensive and practical manual to help health promoters develop their quality assurance strategies and programmes. The manual is intended for both purchasers and providers within the NHS.

Ewles L and Simnett I (1992) *Promoting Health: A Practical Guide*, London, Scutari Press.

Chapters 5 and 6 give further details and a practical guide to Ewles and Simnett's model.

Green LW *et al.* (1980) *Health Education Planning: A Diagnostic Approach*, Mountain View, California, Mayfield Publishing Co.

A detailed account of the PRECEDE model.

Whitehead M and Tones K (1991) *Avoiding the Pitfalls*, London, HEA.

A useful and practical guide to health promotion in different settings.

References

Berry J (1986) "Project health: A step-by-step planning guide for health promotion and preventive medicine programmes", *Health Education Journal*, **45**, 109–111.

Boyd S (1994) M.Sc. health promotion dissertation (unpublished), University of the West of England.

Bristol and District Health Authority and Avon Family Health Services Authority (1993) *The Health of the Nation Strategy for Implementation*, Bristol.

British Standards Institute (1992) *BSI Handbook 22 Quality Assurance*, Milton Keynes, British Standards Institute.

Department of Health (1992) *The Health of the Nation*, London, HMSO.

Evans D, Head M and Speller V (1994) *Assuring Quality in Health Promotion*, Wessex Institute of Public Health Medicine/Health Education Authority.

Ewles L and Simnett I (1992) *Promoting Health: A Practical Guide*, London, Scutari Press.

French J and Milner S (1993) "Should we accept the status quo?", *Health Education Journal*, **52**, 98–101.

Green LW, Kreuter MW, Deeds SFG and Partridge KB (1980) *Health Education Planning: A Diagnostic Approach*, Mountain View, California, Mayfield Publishing Co.

Killoran A (1991) "A healthy start?", *The Health Service Journal*, 29/8/91, 14–16.

Killoran A (1992) *Putting Health into Contracts*, London, HEA.

McCarthy M (1982) *Epidemiology and Policies for Health Planning*, London, King Edward's Hospital Fund for London.

Steel S (1986) *Working in Health Education: A Practical Manual for the Initial Training of Health Education Officers*, HEC/Leeds Polytechnic.

Tannahill A (1990) "Health education and health promotion: planning for the 1990s", *Health Education Journal*, **49**, 194–198.

Tones K (1974) "A systems approach to health education" *Community Health*, **6**, 34–39.

Wright C and Whittington D (1992) *Quality Assurance: An Introduction for Health Care Professionals*, London, Churchill-Livingstone.

13 *Implementing health promotion*

Overview

Key points
The potential for health promotion in different settings:
- Schools and education system
- Workplaces
- Primary health care
- Mass media

The type of health promotion intervention that is adopted will be determined by a range of different factors. These include:

- Identified needs which may relate to a population group, locality or an individual client

- Available resources and staffing

- Your professional remit and expertise.

When considering the range of health promotion interventions, they are usually described in relation to different settings. Settings are used because interventions need to be planned in the light of the resources and organizational structures peculiar to each. Thus health education and promotion takes place, amongst other locations, in:

- Schools and education system

- Workplaces

- Health services particularly primary health care

- Mass media.

Some health promoters prefer to organize their work by focusing interventions on target groups who are felt to have specific and unaddressed needs, for example, young people, older people, Black and ethnic minority groups and women. The value and limitations of targeting have been discussed in Chapter 11 when we looked at the process of needs assessment.

It is also possible to identify different strategies in health promotion such as persuasive communication, community development, policy making and legislative action or behaviour change. We can distinguish strategies such as these from health promotion methods. Methods are specific techniques used in everyday situations and include group discussion, one-to-one counselling and using learning resources. Methods may be used in a variety of different settings and be part of a health promotion strategy (Tones, 1993).

A major theme in this book has been that health promotion is a problematic activity which is influenced by many factors. Health promotion interventions are the result of both practical issues which influence the intervention, and the health promoter's values and beliefs. Depending on the approach or model of health promotion that is favoured, the health promoter will employ a particular type of intervention. For example, those working with a medical model will tend to focus on target groups identified by epidemiological research as having risk factors and seek to effect some change in behaviour. In health service settings, this may be the dominant approach because it is most acceptable and has been part of the health promoter's training. Those who see the most important aim of health promotion as redressing inequalities will use strategies that empower people in community contexts or settings. Beattie's (1991) model of health promotion (see page 95 in Chapter 5) is also useful in illustrating how top-down or bottom-up approaches yield different strategies.

This chapter will look at the types of health promotion interventions that take place in schools, workplaces, primary health care and the mass media. Particular characterisitics of each setting are discussed. Recent policy developments which influence the provision of health promotion are outlined. Examples of innovative practice are given to demonstrate the potential and possibilities of working to promote health.

This chapter is divided into four sections on health promotion in the key settings of:

1. Schools
2. Workplaces
3. Primary health care
4. Mass media.

References

Beattie A (1991) "Knowledge and control in health promotion: a test case for social policy and social theory", in Gabe J, Calnan M and Bury M (eds) *The Sociology of the Health Service*, London, Routledge.

Tones K (1993) "Changing theory and practice: trends in methods, strategies and settings in health education", *Health Education Journal*, **52**, 3.

Part 1: *Health promotion in schools*

Why the school is a key setting for health promotion

School is seen as an important context for health promotion principally because it reaches a large proportion of the population for many years. The emphasis on schools is also a recognition that the learning of health-related knowledge, attitudes and behaviour begins at an early age. The Health Education Authority Primary Schools Project (Williams *et al.*, 1989) has shown that teachers often underestimate the wealth of information young children bring to their learning about health education. Children's perceptions change as they age as do the influences upon them in their health "career". The most effective health education thus takes place as part of an ongoing and progressive programme or spiral curriculum, which builds on previous learning and allows children to extend their knowledge and skills appropriate to their stage of development. The World Health Organisation has described health as a resource for living. We need, therefore, to see education for health as part of all children's entitlement and an essential part of preparation for life.

Reflect on your own experience of health education when you were at school. Do you regard your experience as adequate and appropriate?

? Consider each of the following statements about the aims for health education for young people and indicate whether you agree or disagree.

                                             Agree   Disagree

Health education should:
1. Provide information about how the body works
2. Foster positive personal and social relationships
3. Teach young people to keep fit and feel good
4. Equip young people with the skills to make informed and responsible decisions
5. Inform young people about local services and how to get help
6. Teach young people about the dangers of certain behaviours such as taking drugs
7. Help young people to express their feelings and emotions
8. Teach young people how to say "no"
9. Show young people the wonders of the human body so they don't damage it
10. Put young people off unhealthy behaviour by showing them what can happen
11. Prepare young people for parenthood
12. Be concerned with behaviour and discipline.

Aims for school health education

The development of health education in schools has reflected many approaches to health education and promotion. Health education before the Second World War tended to reflect the medical view of health. Although it was part of teachers' training, it was a fringe subject and almost exclusively concerned with hygiene and fitness. Education in the 1960s saw a swing to being child centred and educational methods sought to develop autonomy and responsibility through discovery learning. Health education emerged as a complex theme of well-being and a state of being human. The Schools Council Health Education Project 5–13 (1977) and Health Education Project 13–18 (1982) saw health education as concerned with making informed decisions and the development of self-esteem. Health themes ranged from the physiological to environmental and community health – a multidimensional view which reflected the holistic concept of the World Health Organisation. Subsequent projects have sought to develop social and lifeskills such as being assertive, making relationships, managing conflict, working in groups and influencing people (Hopson and Scally, 1980, 1982, 1985, 1987; Gray and Hill, 1992; HEA, 1989, 1991). Most health education projects are based on experiential learning. Emphasis is placed on the *process* of education, and finding teaching and learning strategies which encourage reflection and personal awareness. The direction and organization of the health education programme also aims to reflect the needs of the children and young people

In their attempts to build empowerment into education, these projects have sought to raise young people's awareness of inequalities and injustice. However, as Cribb (1986) has pointed out raising young people's expectations about their personal and political efficacy in schools, which are usually hierarchical and authoritarian institutions, may be seen as unethical.

☞ **Key principles of the "My Body Project" (Health Education Council, 1983)**

■ Gaining knowledge with an emphasis on children finding out for themselves
■ Increasing children's ability to make choices about the things that affect their health
■ Promoting self-esteem so children are encouraged to determine for themselves the way they wish to live
■ Providing opportunities for children to consider their attitudes and values.

Alongside the attempts to promote autonomy and decision-making skills are more traditional information-giving approaches. Behind such an approach is the simple assumption that people are rational decision makers whose behaviour will change once they have information about how to live more healthily. Much health education in schools therefore entails the provision of information about the health-damaging effects of certain lifestyles, such as smoking, taking drugs and so on.

Public concern over the health of young people has at times been whipped up into crises over, for example, drug use and sexual activity. From 1986 to 1993 the Department for Education part funded posts in all local education authorities to co-ordinate programmes of drug and sex education which would equip young people with the skills to lead healthy lives. Those appointed as health education co-ordinators recognized that it is not possible to deter young people from health-damaging behaviours and that approaches based on fear are likely to be ineffective (Dorn, 1986).

Guidance on health education in the National Curriculum reflects a view that health is an individual responsibility.

"It is clear that healthy living must be an issue of major importance for everyone, particularly as society can be affected by one health crisis after another. People's health is one of the most important products that any society can create and one of the most important resources required for the creation of any kind of wealth. While everyone is exposed to potential risks to good health, individuals can do much to lessen those risks and to improve the quality of their lives and their environment" (National Curriculum Council, 1990).

The context of health promotion in schools

Section 1 of the 1988 Education Reform Act places a statutory responsibility on schools to provide a broad and balanced curriculum that

- Promotes the spiritual, moral, cultural, mental and physical development of pupils
- Prepares pupils for the opportunities, responsibilities and experience of adult life.

What topics or themes would you expect to find taught in health education in schools?

The National Curriculum for schools includes nine core and foundation subjects. There are also five cross-curricular themes of which health education is one. Although part of the National Curriculum, there is no legal requirement to teach health education. The National Curriculum guidance offers nine components or topic areas for health education:

- Substance use and misuse
- Sex education
- Family life education

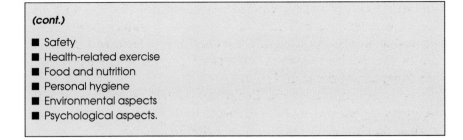

(cont.)

- Safety
- Health-related exercise
- Food and nutrition
- Personal hygiene
- Environmental aspects
- Psychological aspects.

New arrangements for sex education will come into force in September 1994 following the Education Act 1993. These will place a stronger emphasis on a moral framework and family values. All secondary schools will be required to provide sex education and in primary schools this will be discretionary. Parents will have the right to withdraw their children from sex education if they so wish.

The health-promoting school

Health education is not just something which takes place in the curriculum but many aspects of school can be health promoting or health inhibiting. Educationists have long talked of a "hidden curriculum" and the way in which messages can be transmitted through the daily experience of children and young people at school in their surroundings and relationships. For example, the state of many school toilets might suggest that the school does not value hygiene or that the pupils do not require (or deserve) cleanliness and care. Figure 13.1 overleaf shows how many aspects of a school institution can promote health, especially: the physical environment; the nature of relationships between all those in the school; the reciprocal relationship with the community; the quality of the learning experience; the systems of discipline, care and support; and the general ethos of the school.

If education for the health of young people is to focus on more than individual behaviour and be health *promotion*, it needs to acknowledge the influence of the school itself as a health-promoting environment and as part of a wider community.

Limitations and potential of school health education

There has been an encouraging trend towards the strengthening of health education in schools. The number of primary schools with a health education policy has risen from 17% in 1978 to 80% in 1993, and from 68% in secondary schools in 1981 to 89% in 1993 (Lewis, 1993). An HMI report on secondary school inspections between

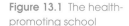

Figure 13.1 The health-promoting school

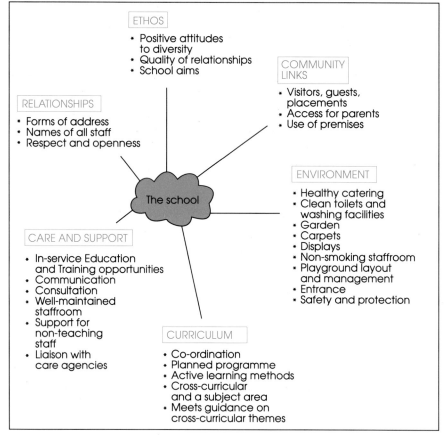

1982 and 1986 found the proportion of schools which made provision for health education has increased from 66% to 92%.

Yet the challenge for schools is to organize this commitment in a coherent way that ensures continuity and progression, and is not merely a response to public and media concerns.

Since the advent of the National Curriculum and regular pupil assessment there has been keen competition for scarce curriculum time. The organizational structures to secure the place of health education are still far from established. In secondary schools a brief timetabled session is the most popular means of giving time to those areas which do not command subject status, such as health education. In primary schools, which still organize the curriulum around topics or integrated themes, health education is rarely included. In both phases, health education may be allied with biology and included as part of science teaching, thus emphasizing the physiological at the expense of the personal and social.

Securing a place for health education will depend on adequate teacher education project. The health education in initial teacher education project (Williams *et al.*, 1990) found few institutions who devoted sufficient time to health education. New arrangements for the training of new teachers by which they will spend 80% of training in the classroom may make it even more difficult to prioritize health education above subject expertise.

Many schools employ outside speakers such as school nurses, health promotion officers or community police officers to deliver sensitive issues which are deemed outside pupils' regular education. Whilst such links with the community should be welcomed, it may mean a greater emphasis on behavioural outcomes. These health promoters are seen as "experts" and therefore encouraged to deliver a top-down health education.

Does health education in schools work?

Demonstrating the effect of health education in schools in isolation from the many other factors that influence health behaviour is extremely difficult. Nevertheless some success has been claimed for smoking education. The "My Body Project", for example, reported gains in knowledge and changes in attitudes, and claimed a probable halving of experimental smoking among 9–13 year olds compared to a control group (Murray *et al.*, 1982). It is more difficult to assess the more broadly based objectives of developing self-esteem and autonomy, or of social and communication skills, which are seen as dimensions of education in general but are also part of self-empowerment in health education. There have been attempts to assess personal and social skills, and for students to complete self-awareness schedules as part of moves to provide students with a broad record of their achievement at school. A recent review of drug prevention education did suggest that lifeskills programmes had resulted in appreciable delays in onset of taking drugs (Dorn and Murji, 1992). It also claimed a consensus that effective health education for young people should be sustained, and is more likely to have impact when it teaches decision making and lifeskills rather than relying on a didactic approach. However, there are too few studies which show whether school-based health education can achieve positive results.

Conclusion

Schools are widely seen as having a key role in health education. This is particularly so when there is public and media concern over health issues. Then the young are seen as a key target population for the provision of information and encouragement of "responsible" attitudes. For example, concern over the spread of HIV infection led the Government in 1991 to include HIV/AIDS education in the statutory National Curriculum for Science. At that time, the provision of sex education was at the discretion of school governing bodies. After intense lobbying by religious groups, HIV education (except its biological aspects) was withdrawn from the National Curriculum in 1994.

Concern over youth crime has led some to call for more emphasis on personal, social and health education, others to call for more religious and moral education, and still others to call for a return to "basics", formal discipline and school uniform, so that would-be truants could be easily identified. Great are the expectations of schools and teachers. Yet we must be realistic and recognize that school-based health education is only one influence on young people's behaviour. It is most likely to be effective where:

- It addresses the needs of young people and starts from where they are in terms of knowledge and experience
- It is supported by an institution which itself is health promoting
- It is supported by health promotion in the community in which young people's health choices are made
- It is delivered by committed and informed teachers with curriculum time and resources which reflect its importance.

Further reading

David K and Williams T (eds) (1987) *Health Education in Schools*, London, Harper and Row.

Although overtaken by changes in school organization and curriculum, this book still provides a wide-ranging view of the school context and argues for an interdisciplinary approach.

Ryder J and Campbell L (1988) *Balancing Acts in Personal, Social and Health Education*, London, Routledge.

Useful for providing an insight into curriculum organization and active learning methods.

Tones K, Tilford S and Robinson Y (1990) *Health Education:*

Effectiveness and Efficiency, London, Chapman & Hall.

Chapter 4 provides an overview of school health education and the evidence for its effectiveness.

Williams T, Roberts J and Hyde H (1990) *Exploring Health Education: A Growth and Development Perspective*, London, HEA/Macmillan.

A short booklet which accompanies the Initial Teacher Education Project. It provides an accessible summary of the stages of children's growth and development and their implications for health education.

References

Cribb A (1986) "Politics and health in the school curriculum", in Rodmell S and Watt A (eds) *The Politics of Health Education*, London, Routledge.

Dorn N (1986) "Can drug education reduce drug experimentation?" *Health at School*, **1**, 66–68.

Dorn N and Murji K (1992) *Drug Prevention: A Review of the English Language Literature*, ISDD Research Monograph 5.

Gray G and Hill F (1992) *Health Action Pack : Health Education for 16–19*, London, HEA/National Extension College.

Health Education Authority (1989) *Health for Life 1 and 2*, London, HEA/Nelson.

Health Education Authority (1991) *Health and Self*, London, HEA/Forbes.

Health Education Council (1983) *My Body*, London, Heinemann.

Hopson B and Scally M (1980,1982,1985,1987) *Lifeskills Teaching Programmes 1,2,3,4*, Leeds, Lifeskills Associates.

Lewis D (1993) "Oh for those halcyon days: a review of school health education over 50 years", *Health Education Journal*, **52**, 3, Autumn.

Murray M, Swan AV, Enock C *et al.* (1982) "The effectiveness of the HEC's My Body school health education project", *Health Education Journal*, **41**, 126–132.

National Curriculum Council (1990) *Curriculum Guidance 5: Health Education*, London, HMSO.

Schools Council/HEC Project (1977) *Health Education 5–13*, London, Nelson.

Schools Council/HEC Project (1982) *Health Education 13–18*, London, Forbes.

Williams T, Wetton N and Moon A (1989) *A Picture of Health*, London, HEA.

Williams T, Roberts J and Hyde H (1990) *Exploring Health Education*, London, HEA/Macmillan.

Part 2: *Health promotion in the workplace*

Why is the workplace a key setting for health promotion?

There are two main reasons for prioritizing the workplace. The workplace gives access to a target group, healthy adults, who are often difficult to reach in other ways. Employees in the workplace are a captive audience for health promotion. Adult men are least likely to come into contact with the health services, so the workplace provides a useful route to reach this group. In 1990, three-quarters of men were economically active compared to just over half of women (Rose, 1993).

The relationship between work and health is complex. In general, attention has focused on the effects of work on health, although it is also acknowledged that poor health will have negative effects on the capacity for paid employment. There is evidence that paid work is good for your health and unemployment can be linked to ill health. Work is beneficial for health because it provides an income, a sense of self-worth, and social networks of colleagues and friends. However, work may also harm health, and most research has concentrated on this aspect of the relationship.

? **Think of a recent work experience.**

- In what ways do you think work contributed to your health?
- In what ways do you think work had a negative impact on your health?
- Overall, would you say work was a positive or a negative influence on your health?

The workplace can affect health in many different ways. Table 13.1 provides a means of classifying these different kinds of relationship.

Hazards tend to be what people think of first when health in the workplace is mentioned. Most legislation is directed towards the containment of hazards and historically safety has always had a higher priority than health. Work which involves handling hazardous or toxic materials may have a direct negative effect on health. Work which provides easy access to hazardous substances is also linked to associated ill health. For example, doctors and pharmacists have high rates of suicide associated with drug overdose.

Table 13.1 The relationship between work and health.

	Direct relationship	Indirect relationship
Hazards	Handling chemicals and toxic materials as part of the job	Job provides access to dangerous drugs
Risky behaviour	Lifting loads and people as part of the job	Excessive drinking associated with work culture
General work environment	Stress generated by work conditions	Lifestyle risk behaviours, e.g. smoking as coping strategy

More often, health is affected through risky behaviour or changed routines. Risky behaviour is the preferred explanation for most official accounts of accidents and injuries sustained in the workplace (Watterson, 1986). This approach extends to the workplace the victim-blaming ideology of some brands of health education. Behaviour which carries health risks may be an integral part of the job or part of the work culture. For example, bartenders have high rates of alcohol-related ill health because drinking heavily is associated with work.

The general work environment and its effects on health is the most neglected dimension. This is due in part to ideological or political reasons, and in part to the fact that such a generalized relationship is hard to research or prove. Because the relationship between work and health is to a large extent indirect, it is often difficult to trace ill health to what happens in the workplace. This in turn leads to the true impact on health from work being underestimated. Focusing on the work environment instead of individual workers' behaviour shifts responsibility on to the employer and has resource implications.

Although the relationship is difficult to quantify, strong evidence implicating the importance to health of the general work environment is becoming available (Theorell, 1991; Sanders, 1993). There is a body of research demonstrating that certain factors associated with some types of work, such as repetitive tasks, lack of autonomy and pressures to meet deadlines, have harmful effects on health (Knox *et al.*, 1985; Johnson *et al.*, 1989). Stress associated with work conditions may lead to the adoption of harmful behaviours as a coping mechanism. Research on smoking shows that nurses smoke more than doctors and that nurses in particularly stressful situations, such as psychiatric units and casualty wards, smoke more than nurses in community settings (Hawkins *et al.*, 1982). So stress related to working conditions may have direct effects on health and may also lead to less healthy lifestyle choices, such as smoking as a way of coping with stress.

What defines the workplace setting?

The relationship between work and health may appear substantial but it is viewed in very different ways by different groups of people. One of the defining characteristics of the workplace setting is that it brings together a variety of groups who have different agendas with regard to work and health. The key parties are: workers or employees and their trade unions or staff associations, employers and managers, occupational health staff, health and safety officers including environmental health officers, and specialist health promoters.

Workers

Workers' organizations have been responsible for some innovative health promotion in the workplace.

 During the 1980s, sexual harassment was raised as a workplace health issue by the white collar union NALGO.

However, the priority of trade unions is defending wages and general working conditions. Membership of trade unions has declined since the mid-1970s, when over half the workforce belonged to trade unions, to 1990, when membership was just under two-fifths (Rose, 1993). So although consultation with unions is an important means of reaching workers, it does not reach everyone. As the key target group, workers need to be fully involved at all stages of the development and implementation of health promotion programmes. Research has shown that effective health promotion programmes are associated with full staff participation (Sanders, 1993).

Employers and managers

Employers and managers have as their first priority the viability of the organization. Health is relevant in so far as it can be shown to be linked to organizational goals. A report of a survey of 41 workplaces found that employers needed to be convinced of hard economic benefits in order to support health promotion (Webb *et al.*, 1988). Examples of hard benefits are: improvements in productivity due to lower rates of sickness, absenteeism and staff turnover; and improved recruitment and retention of trained staff. Soft benefits, such as enhanced corporate image, are also influential. When asked what would enable them to undertake health promotion, employers cited legislation to provide incentives, Government grants, secondment of temporary staff with health promotion skills, and information on effectiveness (Harvey, 1988, Webb *et al.*, 1988).

Occupational health staff

Occupational health staff are employees who provide health services such as first aid, health surveillance, education and advice in large organizations. These services overlap with those provided by the primary health care sector. Over half of Britain's workers and over 80% of workplaces have no access to occupational health services beyond first aid (Webb *et al.*, 1988).

Health and safety officers

Health and safety officers are responsible for ensuring that workplaces conform to safety legislation. They have powers to force workplaces to comply with health and safety regulations, and to impose penalties in the case of non-compliance. Responsibility for workplaces is divided between the Health and Safety Executive and environmental health officers employed by local authorities. Health and safety officers have experienced a reduction in funding together with an increased workload due to the expansion of small businesses and EC legislation.

Health promotion specialists

Health promotion specialists may be involved in health promotion activities in the workplace. They provide a specialist resource for co-ordinating and motivating others to adopt such activities. This service may be provided by NHS departments, voluntary organizations or private companies.

> **?**
>
> **You are a health promoter trying to get workplaces to adopt a CHD prevention programme.**
> What kinds of reasons or evidence would persuade each of the following groups to participate?
>
> ■ Workers
> ■ Managers
> ■ Occupational health staff
> ■ Health and safety officers.

Workers will need to be convinced that the programme concerns their health and is not a covert means of introducing new work practices or conditions, or of using health surveillance to screen employees. Managers will want reassurance that the programme has benefits, preferably economic, for the organization. Occupational health staff will want their professional role to be acknowledged and maintained, and not undermined, by the programme. Health and safety officers will need a clear link to be established between the programme and their role if they are to participate. For example, passive smoking may constitute a health hazard and thus be a suitable topic to address. Above all, the different groups will need to meet to share perspectives and build trusting relationships if such a programme is to be successful.

The involvement of many different groups in workplace health promotion has led to a lack of integrated information. The information that is available is collected by different bodies for specific purposes. For example, statistics on deaths and serious injuries sustained in the workplace is collected by the Health and Safety Executive (HSE), but many cases of work-related ill health go unrecorded. Occupational health staff may have statistics on health checks carried out on staff but this is not generally available. The workplace is characterized by fragmentation of interests and relevant information. This poses obvious difficulties when trying to plan and implement a general health promotion intervention.

The extent of the problem

We have already seen why the ill-health effects of work are likely to be difficult to quantify, leading to under-estimates of the true extent of that effect. Table 13.2 shows that the workplace is implicated in a number of fatal and serious injuries.

It has been estimated that for every one of these accidental deaths in the workplace, there will be another ten deaths from occupational diseases (Schilling, 1984). Fox and Adelstein (1978) calculated that 18% of the variation in mortality between socio-economic groups is occupation related.

This affects the economy as well as people's health. Accidents at work are estimated to cost over £2 billion a year (HSC, 1991).

Background to health promotion in the workplace

Health promotion in the workplace is a relatively new concept, but safety has a much longer history.

> "Employers have long been required to provide safe working conditions. Increasingly they are also recognizing the benefits of a healthy workforce, while trade unions and staff associations are looking for more ways to improve the general health of their membership" (Department of Health 1992, p.25).

Table 13.3 shows some of the key dates of legislation on health and safety in the workplace.

Table 13.2 Injuries at work (adapted from Central Statistical Office, 1993).

	Fatal			Major			Over 3 days*		
	1988/89	1989/90	1990/91	1988/89	1989/90	1990/91	1988/89	1989/91	1990/91
Agriculture, forestry and fishing	46	53	52	583	505	558	1 615	1 626	1 422
Energy and water supply industries	205†	31	27	1 267	1 146	1 074	13 738	11 705	10 276
Total manufacturing industries	101	115	98	7 514	7 497	6 923	56 269	60 154	56 549
Construction	137	154	124	3 660	4 107	3 838	17 566	18 487	18 243
Banking and finance, insurance, business services and leasing	10	10	9	213	277	316	1 183	1 466	1 593
Total reported to enforcement authorities	609	475	433	21 096	21 706	21 222	164 622	167 109	162 888

* Injuries causing incapacity for normal work for more than 3 days.
† Includes injuries from Piper Alpha disaster 6/7/1988

Table 13.3 Key dates in health and safety legislation.

1833	Factory Act	Established Factory Inspectorate with powers to prosecute employers providing unsafe working conditions
1875	Factories and Workshop Act	Centralized Inspectorate; Chief Inspector appointed
1897	Workmen's Compensation Act	Introduced the concept of employer's liability and benefits regardless of who was to blame for accidents
1956	Agriculture Act	Extended legislation to agricultural sector
1972	EMAS	Employment Medical Advisory Service created to give advice and medical monitoring
1974	Health and Safety at Work Act	Placed a legal duty on employers to train, inform, instruct and supervise employees to protect their health and safety Established the Health and Safety Commission (HSC) and the Health and Safety Executive (HSE) which incorporated EMAS
1990	Control of Substances Hazardous to Health (COSHH)	Placed duties on employers to protect employees from the substances they have to work with. Included six key steps: (i) Assessment of risk (ii) Prevention or control of exposure (iii) Use of control measures (iv) Maintenance, examination and testing of control measures (v) Health surveillance (vi) Information, instruction and training
1992	Management of Health and Safety at Work Regulations	Implemented six EEC directives on health and safety at work. Regulations cover: (i) Health and safety management (ii) Work equipment safety (iii) Manual handling of loads (iv) Workplace conditions (v) Personal protective equipment (vi) Display screen equipment

The thrust of recent legislation and policy on health and safety in the workplace has been to rely more on deregulation coupled with tighter specifications of health and safety standards (Harvey, 1988). The employer is responsible for ensuring their workforce is protected from hazards but the enforcement of this is weak. The WHO Target 24 of "Health for All 2000 Europe" (WHO, 1985) states that: "by 1995, people of the region should be effectively protected against work related health risks" and lists four strategies:

■ Occupational health services
■ Development of health criteria
■ Implementation of technical and educational measures
■ Safeguarding the especially vulnerable.

This objective, focusing on protection from risk, is relatively limited. By comparison, the earlier statement of the WHO/International Labour Organisation (1951) defined the aims of occupational health as:

"the promotion and maintenance of the highest degree of physical, mental and social well-being of workers in all occupations by preventing departures from health, controlling risks and the adaptation of work to people and people to their jobs".

?

Think of a workplace you are familiar with.

■ In what ways were people expected to adapt to the job?
■ In what ways was the job adapted to meet the health needs of people?
■ Which approach is preferable, and why?

Health promotion in the workplace is still not widespread. A recent survey found around half of workplaces had provided health promotion programmes (Watson, 1992). Programmes included one-to-one advice and counselling, policy development concerning healthy lifestyles, such as non-smoking policies, and prevention services such as screening. Another survey found health promotion was more likely to be thought important in large workplaces (69%) compared to small workplaces (41%), and that 40% of all workplaces were involved in health promotion during the previous year (HEA, 1993). Compared to other countries, the UK has a low rate of workplace health promotion activities (Philo *et al.*, 1992).

  "Look After Your Heart" (LAYH) is a joint Department of Health/HEA project which was launched in 1988. LAYH provides advice, information and support on healthy lifestyles. It has been adopted by more than 500 employers covering 3.8 million employees.

Workplace health promotion tends to focus on individual lifestyle interventions and neglects environmental or organizational approaches, although both approaches are necessary for maximum effectiveness. This, coupled with a lack of appropriate evaluation of health promotion in the workplace, presents barriers to effective health promotion (Sanders, 1993). However, evidence from the USA demonstrates that health promotion in the workplace is cost effective (Bovell, 1992). Benefits included reduced absenteeism, increased productivity, improved staff attitude and morale, and reduced staff turnover. Where health-promotion interventions have been successful they have had the following features (Sanders, 1993):

- Systematic organization
- Involvement and participation of all staff
- Management support
- Programmes tailored to individual organizations
- Good resourcing
- Long-term interventions.

These findings suggest that there is an untapped potential for health promotion in the workplace programmes.

> **?**   **A workplace CHD prevention programme may include all of the following activities. Which of these have you experienced in your workplace?**
>
> - Planning, implementing and monitoring a smoking policy
> - Provision of a gym and changing rooms
> - Training designated staff in first aid and cardiac resuscitation
> - Introducing healthy menu choices into a staff canteen
> - Provision of a staff counselling service
> - Introduction of lunchtime keep-fit sessions
> - Sending out health education leaflets with pay slips
> - Publicity and events to support "No-Smoking Day"
> - Hosting a mobile cholesterol screening bus for one week
> - Individual fitness testing and suggested activity programmes for staff.

Examples of good practice

>   **The Driver and Vehicle Licensing Authority introduced a two pronged health promotion programme. Staff were given time off work to attend health education courses, and the organization introduced changes such as flexitime, job sharing, child-care facilities, and career break schemes. Sickness absence rates were almost halved between 1985 and 1991** (DVLA, 1989, cited in Sanders, 1993).

> **A weekly yoga and relaxation session held during working hours in the workplace was launched, and ran for 3 months. When compared with a control group, participants' blood pressure was significantly reduced. The difference between the two groups persisted after 4 years of follow-up, even though many participants claimed they no longer practised yoga or relaxation** (Patel et al., 1985).

Conclusion

A body of evidence is becoming available which demonstrates the tangible benefits to be derived from workplace health promotion programmes. Research is also beginning to identify what factors are associated with effective and successful programmes. The challenge now is to increase the coverage of health promotion in the workplace schemes, in terms of both the number of organizations and the scope of the programmes.

Most programmes focus on individual lifestyle advice, monitoring and education. Unless the organizational context is also considered and modified, such programmes are likely to have a limited effect.

Health promotion in the workplace would receive a great impetus if legislation provided incentives to participate. Health promoters can support interventions by facilitating the process of liaison and dialogue amongst all staff. They can also assist by providing specialist input on organizing, planning, implementing and evaluating activities. Tangible benefits need to be demonstrated in order to win managerial support.

Further reading

Health Education Authority (1993) *Health Promotion in the Workplace: A Summary*, London, HEA.

A useful recent summary of workplace health promotion provision.

Sanders D (1993) *Workplace Health Promotion: A Review of the Literature*, Oxford Regional Health Authority.

An excellent recent review of the literature evaluating workplace health promotion programmes in the UK, with comparative data from the USA and Canada. The report focuses on smoking and stress reduction programmes, identifies effective strategies and makes recommendations.

References

Bovell V (1992) "The economic benefits of health promotion in the workplace", in *Action on Health at Work Seminar*, London, HEA.

Central Statistical Office (1993) *Annual Abstract of Statistics 1993*, London, HMSO.

Department of Health (1992) *The Health of the Nation*, London, HMSO.

Fox AJ and Adelstein AM (1978) "Occupational mortality: work or way of life?", *Journal of Epidemiology and Community Health*, **32**, 73–78.

Harvey S (1988) *Just an Occupational Hazard? Policies for Health at Work*, London, King's Fund Institute, Research Report 4.

Hawkins L *et al.* (1982) "Smoking – stress and nurses", *Nursing Mirror*, 13/10/82, 19–22.

Health Education Authority (1993) *Health Promotion in the Workplace: A Summary*, London, HEA.

Health and Safety Commission (1991) *Proposals for Health and Safety (General Provisions) Regulations and Approved Code of Practice: Consultative Document*, Liverpool, Health and Safety Executive.

Johnson J *et al.* (1989) "Combined effects of job strain and social isolation on cardiovascular disease morbidity and mortality in a random sample of the Swedish male working population" *Scandinavian Journal of Work, Environment and Health*, **15**, 271–279.

Knox SS, Theorell T, Svensson JC and Waller D (1985) "The relation of social support and working environment to medical variables associated with elevated blood pressure in young males: a structural model", *Social Science and Medicine*, **21**, 525–531.

Patel C, Marmot MG, Terry DJ, Carruthers M, Hunt B and Patel M (1985) "Trial of relaxation in reducing coronary risk: four year follow-up", *British Medical Journal*, **290**, 1103–1106.

Philo J, Russell J and Pettersson G (1992) *Health at Work: A Needs Assessment in South West Thames Regional Health Authority*, London, SWTRHA.

Rose P (ed.) (1993) *Social Trends 23*, London, Central Statistical Office, HMSO.

Sanders D (1993) *Workplace Health Promotion: A Review of the Literature*, Oxford Regional Health Authority.

Schilling RSF (1984) "More effective prevention in occupational health practice", *Journal of the Society of Occupational Medicine*, **34**, 71–79.

Theorell T (1991) "Health promotion in the workplace", in Badura B and Kickbusch I (eds) *Health Promotion Research: Towards a New Social Epidemiology*, Copenhagen, WHO.

Watson N (1992) *Provision of Employee Health and Welfare Programmes in a Range of Private and Public Sector Organisations in the UK*, University of Sunderland.

Watterson A (1986) "Occupational health and illness: the politics of hazard education", in Rodmell S and Watt A (eds) *The Politics of Health Education: Raising the Issues*, London, Routledge and Kegan Paul.

Webb T, Schilling R, Jacobson B and Babb P (1988) *Health at Work? A Report on Health Promotion in the Workplace*, Research Report No.22, London, HEA.

World Health Organisation (1985) *Targets for Health for All*, Copenhagen, WHO Regional Office for Europe.

World Health Organisation (1951) *Joint ILO/WHO Committee on Occupational Health: Third Report*, Technical Report series No. 135, Geneva, WHO.

Part 3: *Health promotion in primary health care*

What is primary health care?

Primary health care (PHC) refers to the first tier of health provision, provided in local community settings by generalists. PHC

> "... is the first level of contact of individuals, the family and community with the national health system bringing health care as close as possible to where people live, work and constitutes the first element of a continuing health care process" (MacDonald, 1993).

PHC professionals include independent contractors providing NHS care such as general practitioners (GPs) and dentists, as well as staff employed by them such as practice nurses. Other PHC staff, such as health visitors, district nurses and community psychiatric nurses, are employees of health authorities, and social workers are employed by local authorities. Together these professionals make up PHC teams who provide a range of health care services for everybody in the community (see Figure 13.2).

Primary health care provides a setting where health promotion at primary, secondary and tertiary levels takes place. An example of primary prevention, or preventing the occurrence of ill health, is the provision of child immunization services. Secondary prevention is preventing ill health becoming chronic and restoring people to their previous level of health. An example of secondary prevention

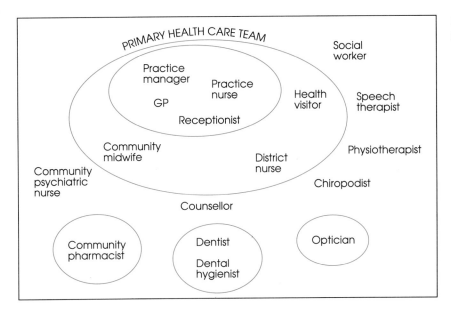

Figure 13.2 Primary health care services

is advising someone with bronchitis to give up smoking. Tertiary prevention, or helping people with chronic or irreversible ill health how to cope with their condition and enjoy their maximum potential for health, is illustrated by the example of asthma clinics which teach people to monitor and manage their condition.

?   **The following activities are all provided in PHC settings.**
Which are examples of primary, secondary and tertiary health promotion?

- Child development checks
- Stroke rehabilitation clubs
- Domiciliary care such as help with getting up and washing
- Asthma clinics
- Dental checks and dental hygiene
- Educating someone with diabetes about managing the condition through diet
- Family planning
- Teaching an insulin-dependent diabetic person how to administer insulin injections
- Well woman clinics
- Advising and supporting an overweight person to lose weight through a calorie-controlled diet and exercise
- Monitoring blood pressure
- Foreign travel vaccinations
- Cancer screening.

Why primary health care is a key setting for health promotion

Primary health care is a key setting because:

- Most people have contact with primary health care practitioners. One study found that over one year 66% of men and 77% women consulted their GP (Ritchie *et al.*, 1981)
- Primary service health promoters have credibility. Research has shown that health professionals working in primary health care enjoy high status and credibility amongst the general public (Table 13.4).

Primary health care has several advantages when compared to the more specialized services provided in the hospital sector. These are:

- Better access because services are provided in the community.
- Improved communication because service users and providers meet on more equal terms. Primary health care providers are generalists. They see people in their own homes as well as in health centres, clinics or surgeries. They see the same people over a number of years and have an understanding of how their health relates to the rest of their lives. These factors help to

break down the barriers between professional and client, and so improve communication.

■ Adequate provision of primary health care services will often mean that more specialized hospital-based services are unnecessary. For example, proper management and monitoring of chronic conditions such as diabetes and asthma should help prevent the development of crises which require hospitalization.

■ Primary health care and prevention is cheaper than hospital care.

Williams *et al.* (1993) suggest prevention is popular with the Government. They cite three factors: the ideological emphasis on individual responsibility; perceived popularity with voters; and perceived economic benefits. The major causes of death such as CHD, stroke, lung cancer, accidents and suicides are to a large extent preventable. Lives lost prematurely through these preventable causes represent an economic loss.

Table 13.4 Credibility of source of health information

Source of information	% respondents who		
	Tend to trust	Tend not to trust	Don't know
Your family doctor	95	4	1
Health visitor/local nurse	87	6	7
HEA booklet or leaflet	83	11	6
Chemist	81	15	3
Poster/leaflet in surgery	70	24	6
TV/radio documentary	63	31	6
Your children working on a health project at school	34	33	30
Newspaper/magazine feature	25	68	7
Friend/neighbour/relative	22	73	5
TV advert	22	73	5

Source: HEC/Consumers' Association, 1983

International and national context

Primary health care has been highlighted as a key setting in both international and national health promotion policies. The WHO "Health for All 2000" programme called for a reorientation of health care services away from the tertiary hospital sector and towards the primary sector:

"The focus of the health care system should be on *primary health care* – meeting the basic health needs of each community through services provided as close as possible to where people live and work, readily accessible and acceptable to all, and based on full community participation" (WHO, 1985, p.5, original emphasis).

The Health of the Nation

The *Health of the Nation* White Paper on health promotion strategy states that:

> "Primary and community health care services will have a major role. Success in Key Areas will depend greatly on the commitment and skills of family and community doctors, nurses, midwives and health visitors, dentists, community pharmacists, opticians and other professionals working in the community" (Department of Health, 1992, p. 35).

Although health promotion is recognized as an intersectoral responsibility requiring input from many different agencies, the lead role of the NHS is acknowledged:

> "The role of the health professions – and indeed everyone who provides health care and related services – will be crucial to the success of the strategy. Their opportunities to help and advise individuals, families and communities are unparalleled" (Department of Health, 1992, p.30).

A training manual, *Better Living, Better Lives*, has been issued by the Department of Health (1993) to all GP practices, with the aim of supporting activity to achieve the "Health of the Nation" targets.

General practice

GPs are being encouraged to become budget holders in charge of their own funds. One offshoot of this is that some GP practices are starting to employ complementary therapists such as acupuncturists, herbalists, counsellors and hypnotists.

The new funding arrangements for GPs are also of vital importance in shifting the focus from cure to prevention. From 1 July 1993, GP practices have had a new system of funding for their health promotion work. There are three funding levels or bands, from the lowest band 1 to the highest band 3.

Band 1: programme to reduce smoking through establishing an age sex register, collecting information on the smoking habits of patients, and offering advice, interventions and follow-up.

Band 2: the above plus a programme to minimize mortality and morbidity from coronary heart disease (CHD), hypertension and stroke. This is to be achieved by opportunistic checks to discover raised blood pressure, maintenance of a register of patients with hypertension, CHD and stroke, and lifestyle interventions for these patients.

Band 3: the above plus a primary CHD and stroke prevention programme which includes the following: collecting information on risk factors, monitoring risk factors, offering lifestyle advice, other interventions and follow-up, and focusing activity on priority groups including non-attenders.

Targets in terms of practice population coverage are set for each of these activities. It is also stated that all activity should involve other people and agencies. There are additional payments for chronic disease management programmes for asthma and diabetes. This funding arrangement replaces the open-ended commitment to fund health promotion clinics run by GPs. Whilst there were criticisms of the clinic payment system, it has also been argued that the new arrangements are restrictive and focus on CHD to the exclusion of everything else:

> "Smear, contraception and well woman health checks are important but are not being prioritized by Government. The balance was better before" (Orme, 1993).

The new GP contract states that registered adult patients should be offered a health check every 3 years, regardless of health status. Those patients aged 75 or over should be visited and receive a health check every year. It is not certain whether this additional workload is feasible or even desirable.

Although GPs figure so prominently in Government funding of health promotion, they themselves are less wholehearted about their role in health promotion in PHC. A recent survey of GPs [General Services Medical Committee/British Medical Association, (GSMC/BMA), 1992] found a general sense of low morale, with four-fifths of respondents agreeing that their role within the NHS is undervalued and that too much is being asked of general practice at the present. In this context, the health promotion role of GPs comes under question:

> "The preventive role of the GP is overdone. GPs aren't experts on diet and exercise. A lot of health problems are due to poverty and homelessness – that's a political problem not a GP's" (Orme, 1993).

Half the respondents agreed that more effort and resources should be devoted to health promotion by the NHS, but 70% did not think that screening healthy people saves resources (GSMC/BMA, 1992). Research supports this scepticism, and has found that the inverse care law, whereby those who stand to benefit most have the lowest take-up rates of services, operates in respect of health checks (Blaxter, 1984; Crombie, 1984).

Nurses

Much of the health promotion practised in PHC settings is carried out by nurses. Practice nurses, health visitors, midwives, district nurses and community psychiatric nurses have much scope for health education in their daily contact with the practice population. Much of this is opportunistic, and a recent survey found that three-fifths of practice nurses felt they needed more training in how to plan and organize health promotion (Calnan, 1992). Nurses are also responsible for collecting information on patients' health status and for health surveillance. Pilot projects have demonstrated the potential for community nurses to work in group and community settings to empower clients (Drennan, 1986). However, the demands of their statutory duties and caseload size mean these types of health promotion activities tend to take a low priority.

 Pennywell Neighbourhood Centre in Sunderland opened in 1990. The centre aims to provide a multiagency community development approach to health for people living on the estate. The centre provides a broad range of child care, primary health and community support services. Health visitors run several health clinics, and other activities include a safety equipment loan scheme, a women's group, and training in first aid and creche work. The centre's work is being evaluated.

Family Health Services Authorities (FHSAs)

FHSAs in addition to administering payments to GPs, dentists, opticians and pharmacists also provide training, education and support for health promotion practice in PHC.

Care in the community

The Care in the Community Act, in operation since 1993, also impacts upon primary health services. The new legislation requires social services departments and health authorities to liaise together to provide individualized care programmes for people in need.

Planned or opportunistic health promotion?

Policy planning and implementation seeks to build health promotion into PHC, replacing previous health promotion interventions which were largely opportunistic, *ad hoc*, and unplanned.

A recent review of research investigating smoking cessation interventions concluded that:

". . . advice from GPs is more effective than no advice. On average, 5% of smokers will stop smoking, and stay abstinent for at least a year, following brief advice from a GP during one consultation. . . The effectiveness can be increased by offering smokers literature on smoking, negotiating a date to stop smoking and making a contract with the smoker to stop on this date, and offering follow-up appointments to deal with problems in stopping smoking" (Sanders, 1992, p.11).

This example illustrates the advantages of opportunistic health education, but there are also disadvantages.

You may have included some of the following:

How many advantages and disadvantages of opportunistic health education can you identify?

■ Opportunistic health education relies on the decisions of individual practitioners. This leads to patchy and uneven implementation, on a basis of chance rather than proven need.

■ Health promotion remains a marginalized luxury, to be tacked on at the end of a consultation if there is time. Research has shown that lack of time is an important factor limiting the amount of health promotion undertaken by both GPs and nurses (Littlewood and Parker, 1992; Tapper-Jones *et al.*, 1990).

■ Doubts as to the value of opportunistic health education have been expressed. Almost half the community nurses in one study thought that raising the subject of smoking with patients consulting for unrelated problems made them annoyed (Littlewood and Parker, 1992).

The advantages of opportunistic health promotion include:

■ Immediate relevance of information
■ Highly motivated patients
■ The ability to adapt and modify the input to suit individual needs.

The emphasis of recent policy has been on developing more planned and proactive health promotion activities. Health surveillance and targeted health information and advice to patients with recognized lifestyle risk factors has emerged as the most favoured strategy. CHD, the major cause of premature death, has been identified as the priority health topic. It has not been established that such an approach will be effective in preventing ill health. Indeed, given the evidence on the social causes of ill health (see Chapter 2), such an individualized approach is problematic. The focus on CHD is also debatable. Whilst CHD is a major health problem, it is also true that a significant amount of GP work is related to mental ill health and other aspects of physical health (see Table 13.5).

Examples of good practice

We have described the current policy context for health promotion in primary health care as being somewhat limiting. However, this has not prevented PHC staff from setting up many innovative projects around the country. The following examples of good practice demonstrate the variety and potential of health promotion in primary health care.

Table 13.5 General practice consultation rates by selected diagnostic groups.

Diagnostic group	% GP consultations
Diseases of respiratory system	19
Mental disorders	10
Diseases of circulatory system	8
Diseases of nervous system and sense organs	7
Diseases of musculoskeletal system	7
Diseases of skin and subcutaneous tissue	6
Diseases of digestive system	5
Diseases of genito-urinary system	5

Source: Royal College of GPs 1970/71 National Morbidity Survey, cited in Royal College of General Practitioners (1979).

The Khush Dil Happy Heart Express Project is based in inner city Birmingham and liaises with the multicultural community to promote a coronary protective diet. Activities include a mobile caravan for practical cook and taste sessions, and general health discussions as well as liaison with shopkeepers and food manufacturers to promote healthy foods.

A number of districts in the North West Thames Region have established district nursing schemes to reach homeless people. Kensington, Chelsea, Westminster and Brent district nursing services are provided in hostels and day centres for the homeless, and they will also see people who refer themselves. West London provides nursing services in night shelters.

National organizations such as the HEA Primary Health Care Unit based in Oxford provide centralized support for health promotion in PHC.

The primary health care facilitator role was piloted in Oxford and is now a national project. PHC facilitators are located in district health authorities and family health service authorities, and act as catalysts for the development and support of health promotion and preventive services.

Typical activities include:

- Providing training for practice nurses
- Promoting healthy alliances through liaison and networking
- Developing resources for use in PHC
- Developing common guidelines and policies for care.

"Helping People Change" is a health promotion training and resources programme for primary health care professionals. It is provided by the PHC Unit of the Health Education Authority and adopts a cascade training model. A "train the trainers" course is available at

> **(cont.)**
>
> **regional level. Participants are then encouraged to train other PHC professionals in their district. The aim of the project is to give PHC professionals the skills, knowledge and attitudes to:**
>
> ■ Understand the concept of risk management
> ■ Understand the process of change and how to intervene effectively
> ■ Apply these principles to make brief health promotion interventions.

Conclusion

Policy initiatives such as the *Health of the Nation* (Department of Health, 1992) and the new GP funding arrangements represent a significant step forward. Health promotion is now firmly on the NHS agenda. However, by channelling funding into certain topics and strategies, the new emphasis on health promotion has also led to certain constraints in practice. CHD has been selected as the primary topic, and individual lifestyle advice, surveillance and monitoring have been the strategies chosen for funding. Other strategies, such as community development work, have not been legitimized in the same way. This has not prevented the development of many examples of innovative practice which seek to maximize health promotion within the PHC setting.

Research suggests that the different health professionals in PHC have different perceptions as to what constitutes health promotion and the degree to which it is effective. GPs have been targeted as health promoters by the Government, yet they remain unconvinced of the value and feasibility of their efforts.

An integrated team approach is a vital first step in shifting PHC from treatment to prevention. Pooling information about the effectiveness of health promotion in PHC is also important, and the HEA PHC Unit has taken a lead in this.

Further reading

Department of Health (1993) *Better Living, better Lives*, London, HMSO.

This manual to accompany **The Health of the Nation** *gives detailed advice and information on how to implement a CHD prevention programme in PHC.*

References

Blaxter M (1984) "Equity and consultation rates in general practice", *British Medical Journal*, **288**, 1963–1967.

Calnan M and Williams S (1992) "The role of general practitioners in coronary heart disease prevention in primary health care", a study commissioned by the Department of Health, London.

Crombie DL (1984) "Social class and health status: inequality or difference", *Journal of the Royal College of General Practitioners*, Occasional Paper 25.

Department of Health (1992) *The Health of the Nation*, White Paper London, HMSO.

Department of Health (1993) *Better Living, Better Lives*, London, HMSO.

Drennan V (1986) *Effective Health Education in the Inner City*, London, Paddington and North Kensington Health Authority.

General Medical Services Committee/British Medical Association (1992) *Your Choices for the Future: A Survey of GP Opinions: A UK Report*, Electoral Reform Ballot Services.

Health Education Council/ Consumer's Association (1983) *General Household Survey*.

Littlewood J and Parker I (1992) "Community nurses' attitudes to health promotion in one regional health authority", *Health Education Journal*, **51**, 87–89.

MacDonald J (1993) *Primary Health Care – Medicine in its Place*, London, Earthscan.

Orme J (1993) *Health Promotion in Primary Health Care: Bands or Boundaries*, MSc dissertation, University of the West of England.

Ritchie J, Jacoby A and Bone M (1981) *Access to Primary Health Care*, London, HMSO.

Royal College of General Practitioners (1979) *Morbidity Statistics from General Practice 1971–2. Second national study*, London, HMSO.

Sanders D (1992) *Smoking Cessation Interventions: Is Patient Education Effective?* Department of Public Health and Policy, London School of Hygiene and Tropical Medicine.

Tapper-Jones L, Smail S, Pill R and Davis R (1990) "Doctors' attitudes towards patient education in the primary care consultation", *Health Education Journal*, **49**, 47–50.

Williams SJ, Calnan M, Cant SL and Coyle J (1993) "All change in the NHS? Implications of the NHS reforms for primary care prevention", *Sociology of Health and Illness*, **15**, (1), 43–67

World Health Organisation (1985) *Targets for Health for All*, Copenhagen, WHO Regional Office for Europe.

Part 4: *Using the mass media in health promotion*

The use of mass media in health promotion has a long history.

> ☛ In 1603 James 1, King of England, proclaimed that smoking is: "A custom, lothesome to the eye, hateful to the Nose, harmful to the braine, dangerous to the Lungs and in the black stinking fume thereof, neerest resembling the horrible Stigian smoke of the pit that is bottomelesse . . . by the immoderate taking of tobacco, the wealth of a great number of people is impaired and their bodies unfit for labour."

The powerful effects of propaganda during the Second World War were influential in persuading health promoters to adopt a similar strategy. In 1953 John Burton, the editor of the *Health Education Journal*, stated that:

> "The first 10 years of our existence could well be called the era of propaganda. Health education has been realized mainly in terms of mass publicity on all fronts. *Ad hoc* exhortations have been directed at the public following closely the patterns of commercial advertising. In addition much energy and ingenuity has been expended on exhibitions and displays of all kinds, and even on carnivals" (Burton, cited in Tones, 1993, p.128).

However, by this time there had already developed a concern that such a strategy was not working or delivering the goods and that the role of the mass media in health promotion needed to be redefined:

> "Many (have come) to feel that mass publicity methods were expensive and relatively ineffective in changing people's health habits and beliefs, and that health education would have to be planned on a more personal basis" (Burton, cited in Tones, 1993, p.128).

Today we are further down the road of identifying what the mass media can and cannot achieve in health promotion. However, the high profile of the mass media continues to make it a popular choice politically. Advertising in the mass media is a central strategy in the Government's AIDS prevention programme and an important element in many other major campaigns.

Definitions

Mass media: any printed or audio-visual material designed to reach a mass audience. This includes newspapers, magazines, radio, television, billboards, exhibition displays, posters and leaflets.

Message: a cultural communication encoded in signs and symbols.

Marketing: the sum total of all activities (the marketing mix) designed to persuade people to adopt certain behaviours.

Advertising: one component of the marketing mix.

Audience segmentation: The division of a mixed population into more homogeneous groups or market segments. Market segments are defined by certain shared characteristics which affect attitudes, beliefs and knowledge. Targeting specific market segments allows for more specific messages which will have a greater effect.

History of the mass media in health promotion

Early optimism that the mass media could induce massive shifts in attitudes or behaviour has not proved to be realistic. The view of the mass media as a hypodermic syringe having an immediate and direct effect on the audience has been replaced by the aerosol spray analogy:

> "...we now begin to look at mass communication as a sort of aerosol spray. As you spray it on the surface, some of it hits the target: most of it drifts away; and very little of it penetrates" (Mendelsohn, 1968).

Gatherer *et al.* (1979) looked at 49 evaluated studies of mass media campaigns and found mixed evidence of effectiveness. Small short-term increases in knowledge in the order of 6% were reported. Attitudes did shift to some extent but not necessarily in the desired direction. There was great variability in behavioural outcomes, ranging from no change to a maximum of long-term change in the order of 10%.

In the light of unrealistically high expectations these results have been viewed as failures. Yet this is not necessarily the case. It is the expectations which need reassessment, in order to establish what are reasonable criteria for success when using the mass media. Three main factors need to be re-examined: the nature of mass media coverage and its impact on the audience; the role of advertising within a marketing strategy; and the role of specific training and expertise in using the mass media.

The nature of mass media and its effects

That mass media reach a wide audience is considered to be a major advantage. However, there are also more negative implications of this fact. The media are cultural communications which are indirect, leaving scope for different interpretations or readings of the same content.

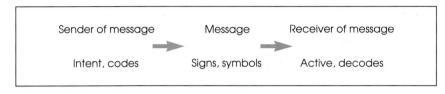

| Sender of message | Message | Receiver of message |
| Intent, codes | Signs, symbols | Active, decodes |

Figure 13.3 Media messages.

Messages are coded into signs and symbols which have meaning within specific codes. The message is encoded by the sender, and decoded by the receiver (see Figure 13.3). The intention is that messages should be decoded and understood according to the intentions of the sender; but there is ample opportunity for messages to be decoded in different ways, as the example below illustrates.

> **?**
>
> **In 1986 and 1987 the Government launched a major media campaign on AIDS, including a leaflet delivery to all households. One advertisement featured a picture of an iceberg with the slogan "Don't die of ignorance".**
>
> ■ How many possible interpretations of this advertising illustration and slogan are there?
> ■ What do you think was the intended message?
> ■ Do you think this message was successfully communicated?

The intention was that people should recognize that HIV infection is preventable, be motivated to acquire correct information on prevention and practise safer sex. However, many people connected the ominous picture of icebergs and the word "die" with HIV/AIDS. This reinforced their belief that sex, death and HIV are related but also raised anxiety levels. Knowledge increased, but so too did people's perception of their own behaviour as low risk (perhaps as a means of dealing with their anxiety), making it unlikely that they would change their behaviour (Wober, 1988). It is in the nature of mass media that there is no immediate feedback, so messages which are decoded in ways not intended may survive and become reinforced through repetition or repeated exposure.

Although the mass media reaches a mass audience, it typically addresses people as individuals. Messages tend to be more meaningful and effective the more targeted they are, but to target certain groups carefully means the message will have less impact on other groups. The benefits of a mass audience need to be balanced against the benefits of closer targeting and a balance struck between the two opposing pressures.

It is important to understand how the mass media influences audiences, if effective use is to be made of this strategy. Glover (1984) proposes four models of this relationship:

1. Hypodermic syringe

This model, discussed above, assumes a passive audience who can be swayed by a manipulative mass media. It was given credibility by the assumed power of wartime propaganda.

 In 1938 Orson Welles broadcast a radio version of H.G. Wells' classic science fiction story *The War of the Worlds*. Thousands of American listeners assumed the story of an imminent alien invasion from outer space was real, and panic spread as people tried to flee (Cantril, 1958).

This model has since been discredited, and a view of audiences as more active and selective has developed. However, the belief that the media are inherently persuasive and influential remains popular. For example, in the run up to a general election, political parties use public media broadcasts to try and win votes.

2. Two-step flow model

This suggests that effective mass media works in stages. Key opinion leaders are active members of an audience who are influenced by the media. These opinion leaders then transmit to other people (passive members of an audience) through inter-personal means of communication (Katz and Lazarsfeld, 1955). This model has been criticized as too simplistic and rejected.

3. Uses and gratifications

This suggests that individual members of an audience are active in accepting some communications and rejecting others. People use the media to meet their own individual needs.

4. Cultural effects model

The media are seen as playing a key role in creating the beliefs and values which people use to make sense of their society. This model acknowledges the importance of social groups and communities in generating beliefs and cultures. The media address people not as individuals but as members of identifiable groups, and media content is filtered and interpreted through cultural norms.

A person's views on the media and how they should be used, regulated and controlled is linked to their view of how the media operates.
Which of the four models outlined above are suggested by these headlines?

- Youth in alleged copycat attack after watching video
- Nine o'clock threshold flouted by trailers
- Soft porn a useful means of sublimation, claims psychologist
- Feminists lobby parliament to ban pornography
- Tobacco sponsorship of televised sport makes a mockery of voluntary agreement
- Cable brings deregulated viewing to thousands – just pay for the channels you want
- Media responsible for Labour poll defeat.

Media coverage of health issues tends to favour certain types of stories over others. Karpf (1988) identifies four "preferred frameworks" for health coverage. These are:

1. Medical dominance, e.g. stories of miracle cures, surgery and high-technology interventions, based in hospitals and featuring doctors
2. Consumerism, e.g. self-help stories of how to choose and obtain health services.
3. "Look after Yourself", e.g. health education messages about changing to healthier lifestyles.
4. Social, political and environmental, e.g. health implications of policy change or how the environment affects health. This is the least popular framework.

The media may be ineffective in putting across explicit health promotion messages but implicitly powerful messages about health are conveyed. For example, there is a tendency towards sensationalism in the media, which is seen as the key to gaining audiences. So personalities, disasters, scandals and miracle cures are seized upon. This affects all media but especially the "tabloid" newspapers, which have a lower social class readership. It has been argued that the more sensational and less informative nature of health coverage in the tabloids, when compared to the "quality" newspapers, constitutes yet another health inequality (Research Unit in Health and Behaviour Change, 1989).

Entertainment programmes often convey implicit messages about health behaviour. For example, alcohol is shown in many fictional programmes as a useful social lubricant (Hansen, 1986). Smoking is less often seen in TV fiction as it becomes less acceptable and a minority behaviour in society. Soap operas are a powerful vehicle for health messages. Through their characters, soaps can explore the causes and motivating factors underlying people's adoption of certain health behaviours.

> **?** **Think of characters who smoke in soap operas. Are they 'good' characters? Or bad?**
> ■ How many programmes use the pub as a central focus?

A further factor to take into account when using the media is the advertising of many products which impact upon health and the extent to which media survival depends upon this source of revenue. This dependence may affect or compromise the media's coverage of health issues. For example, health coverage is quite extensive in women's magazines but smoking is seldom addressed. Tobacco advertising is an important source of income for such magazines (Amos, 1984).

Advertising, marketing and the mass media

McCron and Budd (1981) argue that the unrealistic expectations of media effectiveness were due in part to a basic misunderstanding. Health promoters assumed that advertising alone was responsible for the behaviour change achieved by commercial companies. They failed to appreciate that advertising is just one part of what is called "the marketing mix", which is a whole range of strategies used to sell products to people.

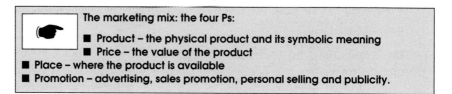

> ☞ **The marketing mix: the four Ps:**
> ■ **Product – the physical product and its symbolic meaning**
> ■ **Price – the value of the product**
> ■ **Place – where the product is available**
> ■ **Promotion – advertising, sales promotion, personal selling and publicity.**

In addition, advertising a commercial product is very different from trying to sell health. Advertising typically mobilizes existing predispositions, whereas health promotion typically tries to counter them. For example, advertising associates the product (e.g. beer, crisps) with something people desire, such as fun. All too often, health education messages are about not indulging, and therefore by implication, not having fun (e.g. don't drink and drive, eat less fat).

Advertising is selling things in the here and now, to be immediately consumed and enjoyed. By contrast, health education messages are often about foregoing present enjoyment for future benefits (see Figure 13.4). Advertising spends large sums of money for relatively small shifts in behaviour. Health education spends a fraction of commercial budgets attempting to generate large shifts in behaviour.

 In 1988 tobacco companies spent over £100 million on promoting tobacco. The HEA's total budget for that year was around £10 million.

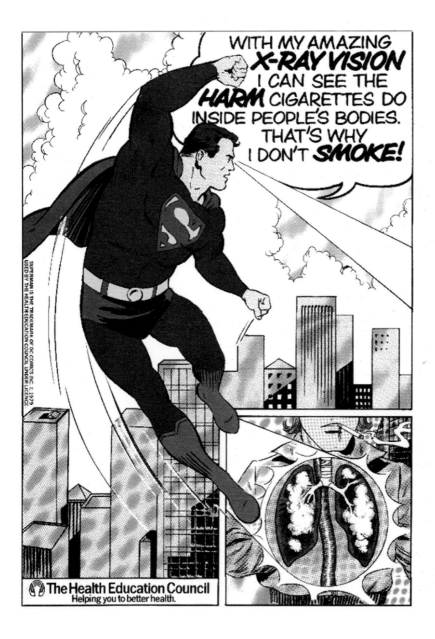

Figure 13.4 Superman and Nick O'Teen. Source: Health Education Authority.

The need for media training

Health promoters have been rather slow to appreciate that maximizing media coverage requires specialist skills and training. One report discovered a number of lost opportunities when media coverage could have been helpful and identified some of the contributory factors (South East Thames Regional Health Promotion Group, 1981). Health promoters avoided the media due to fear of misrepresentation, arguing that no coverage is preferable to inaccurate coverage. They were nervous of being interviewed because they felt they had to have all the facts before going public. A further obstacle was the need for many employees to have official clearance before any contact with the media.

If health promoters are to take a more active role themselves, they need training in presentation skills and how to get the message across, given the time and space constraints. Such training might include networking skills, writing press releases, interviewing skills, and designing effective posters, leaflets and audio-visual aids. This in turn would enable use of the media to become a more effective and widespread health promotion strategy.

What the mass media can and cannot do

Research and evaluation of the use of the mass media in health promotion has led to a reassessment of its potential and limitations (RUHBC, 1989, Tones *et al.*, 1990; Tones, 1993). It is now accepted that the mass media can:

- raise consciousness about health issues
- help place health on the public agenda
- convey simple information
- change behaviour if other enabling factors are present.

Factors which enable behaviour change include: existing motivation, supportive circumstances and advocating simple one-off behaviour change (e.g. carry a donor card).

Using the media is more effective if:

- It is part of an integrated campaign including other elements such as one-to-one advice.
- The information is new and presented in an emotional context
- The information is seen as being relevant for "people like me".

The mass media cannot:

- Convey complex information
- Teach skills
- Shift people's attitudes or beliefs. If messages are presented which

challenge basic beliefs, it is more likely that the message will be ignored, dismissed, or interpreted to mean something else.
- Change behaviour in the absence of other enabling factors.

☞ **"No Smoking Day" is a major annual health promotion event which has been running since 1984. Its aims are to:**

- Encourage and assist smokers to give up for the day
- To bring the day to the attention of as many people as possible
- To involve as many people as possible in activities related to smoking education
- In the long term, assist those wishing to give up smoking to do so for good

The campaign has a budget of £400,000. Its strategy is two-fold: a public relations campaign and supporting local organizers. Ten per cent of the budget is allocated to research and evaluation. The event is evaluated by quantitive survey data and qualitative research into local activities. Evaluation of the 1989 "Day" found:

- High prompted awareness of the campaign (86%)
- 19% smokers claimed to have tried to participate in the "Day", of which 41% claimed to have quit for the whole day
- Three months later, 0.5% smokers had quit and were still not smoking.

Source: McGuire, 1992.

Conclusion

Health promotion in the mass media takes many different forms including advertising, information and role modelling. A health education leaflet and a 30 second advertisement for a national health promotion programme are both examples of the use of mass media in health promotion. There is now a body of research evidence documenting the potential and limitations of mass media as a strategy in health promotion. Alongside this has developed an awareness of how to use the mass media more effectively, and an acknowledgement that specialist training is needed in order to access and use the media to its full potential. However, using the media is not merely a matter of technique. Using the media means entering into a system of codes and meanings which may run counter to the message being promoted.

? **Feminists have argued that the media and advertising maintain and reproduce sexist stereotypes of women. These stereotypes concentrate on women's physical appearance and their relationship to men. The representation of women in these ways is "unhealthy" because it denies their autonomy.**

- Do you think health education materials portray women as autonomous?
- Is it possible to represent women in the media in 'healthy' ways?

Further reading

Leathar DS, Hastings GB and Davies JK (eds) (1981) *Health Education and the Media, Vol. 1* Oxford, Pergamon Press.

Leathar DS and O'Reilly KM (eds) (1986) *Health Education and the Media*, Vol. 2, Oxford, Pergamon Press.

Two edited volumes which present a range of research examining the use of the media in health promotion.

Research Unit in Health and Behavioural Change (1989) *Changing the Public Health*, Chichester, John Wiley and Sons.

Chapter 4 is a useful summary and review of the use of mass media in health promotion.

Siddall S (1982) *Getting the Message Across*, Bristol, Farren.

A useful and practical guide to designing health education materials.

Tones K, Tilford S and Robinson Y (1990) *Health Education: Effectiveness and Efficiency*, London, Chapman & Hall.

Includes detailed accounts of evaluated mass-media campaigns.

References

Amos A (1984) "Women's magazines and smoking", *Health Education Journal*, **43**, 45–50.

Cantril H (1958) "The invasion from Mars", in Maccoby EE, Newcomb TM and Hartley EL (eds) *Readings in Social Psychology*, New York, Henry Holt.

Gatherer A, Parfit J, Porter E and Vessey M (1979) *Is Health Education Effective?*, London, Health Education Council.

Glover D (1984) *The Sociology of the Mass Media*, Ormskirk, Causeway Press.

Hansen (1986) "The portrayal of alcohol on television", *Health Education Journal*, **45**, (3), 127–131.

Karpf A (1988) *Doctoring the Media*, London, Routledge and Kegan Paul.

Katz E and Lazarsfeld P (1955) *Personal Influence: the Part Played by People in the Flow of Mass Communication*, Glencoe, Illinois, Free Press.

McCron R and Budd J (1981) "The role of the mass media in health education: an analysis", in Meyer M (ed.) *Health Education by Television and Radio*, Munich, KG Saur.

McGuire C (1992) *Pausing for Breath: A Review of No Smoking Day Research 1984–1991*, London, HEA.

Mendelsohn H (1968) "Which shall it be: mass education or mass persuasion for health?", *American Journal of Public Health*, **58**, 131–137.

Research Unit in Health and Behavioural Change (1989) *Changing the Public Health*, Chichester, John Wiley and Sons.

South East Thames Regional Health Promotion Group (1981) *Getting Through*, London.

Tones K, Tilford S and Robinson Y (1990) *Health Education: Effectiveness and Efficiency*, London, Chapman & Hall.

Tones K (1993) "Changing theory and practice: trends in methods, strategies and settings in health education", *Health Education Journal*, **52**, 126–139.

Wober JM (1988) "Informing the British public about AIDS", *Health Education Research*, **3**, 19–24.

Evaluation in health promotion 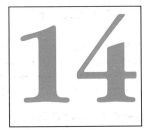 14

Overview

The growth of health promotion as a discipline has been accompanied by discussion of the role of evaluation in this process and attempts to define its meaning. Alongside this theoretical debate concerning the role and function of evaluation there has developed a practical discussion of "how to do it". This chapter is mainly concerned with the first issue. We start by considering why it is important to evaluate and how to define evaluation. Different types of evaluation are identified and discussed, including process, impact and outcome evaluation. Performance indicators are defined, and their use in monitoring and evaluation considered. The case for pluralistic evaluation is examined. Common dilemmas facing the health promoters who wish to evaluate their work are then considered, including: deciding what to measure, being sure that results are due to the health promotion input, when to evaluate, knowing what constitutes success, and deciding whether evaluation is worth the effort.

> **Key points**
> - The three Es: Efficiency, Effectiveness and Economy
> - Process, impact and outcome evaluation
> - Performance indicators
> - Pluralistic evaluation
> - Dilemmas in evaluation

Does health promotion work?

Health promotion is often thought to be a vague activity where it is difficult to demonstrate success. This is not the case. As a relatively new discipline, health promotion has been expected to prove itself according to rigorous, or in some instances unrealistic, criteria. Yet the overwhelming weight of evidence is that health promotion *does* work. Three surveys of health promotion interventions concluded that the majority of health promotion interventions are effective (Gatherer *et al.*, 1979; Bell *et al.*, 1985; Green and Lewis, 1986). Gatherer *et al.* (1979) found that 85% of 62 studies reported improved knowledge levels, 65% of 39 studies reported changed attitudes in the desired direction, and 75% of 123 studies reported behavioural change.

> ☛ The North Karelia Project launched in 1971 was a heart disease prevention project located in an area in Finland which had the highest rate of premature deaths from coronary heart disease in Europe. The project used an integrated community-wide approach which included the mass media, the development of a schools programme, use of volunteers to act as lay educators and role models in the community, and the production of low-fat foods. Evaluation showed that risk behaviours, such as fat consumption and smoking, declined more dramatically in North Karelia than in the rest of Finland. This change in behaviour was matched by a reduction in risk factors for CHD, such as mean serum cholesterol and blood pressure, which again was greater than for the rest of Finland. The population reported improvements in their health and general well-being. There was a greater reduction in the death rate from CHD in North Karelia than for Finland as a whole.
>
> Source: Tones et al., 1990.

Why evaluate health promotion activities?

Evaluation is a complicated process and uses resources which might otherwise be used for programme planning and implementation. What is the justification for using scarce resources to evaluate? Evaluation is needed to ensure that health promotion activities are having the intended effects. Health promotion is an uncertain business and there are no guarantees that certain effects will follow certain inputs. Evaluation is needed to assess results and to determine if objectives have been met.

The professional development of health promotion practice depends on evaluation. Evaluating activities helps inform future plans and contributes to the building up of a knowledge base for health promotion. It also helps prevent the reinvention of the wheel, by informing other health promoters of the effectiveness of different methods and strategies. Health promotion has at its disposal a large repertoire of methods, each of which has its own adherents and publicists. It is only through evaluation of different strategies and approaches that the health promoter is able to make informed choices about which methods to use and when. Evaluation is a necessary component of the reflective practitioner and enhances job satisfaction.

Evaluation is necessary to the ongoing survival and viability of health promotion. To compete successfully for resources in today's economic climate, health promoters must be able to demonstrate hard results. It is not enough to have good intentions. Evaluation of activities is necessary to win credibility and status for health promotion. This issue is perhaps most acute in health promotion services located within the NHS, where the standard against which health promotion must prove itself is that of scientific medicine. Although it can be argued that many medical procedures are adopted for widespread use without proven efficacy (Cochrane,

1972), alternative approaches to health (including health promotion) are often required to prove themselves according to scientific standards. It is partly as a result of these pressures that quantitive outcome evaluation has been preferred over process evaluation.

Evaluation may also be used to determine the efficiency, or extent to which aims and objectives are met, of different methods. This information may be used to help decide the best use of limited resources.

> **?** **A health promotion unit uses two different methods to encourage dietary change – intensive groupwork and a mass media campaign. The primary objective is to reduce fat consumption. The groupwork participants reduce their fat intake by 7% whereas the mass media audience reduce their fat intake by 3%.**
>
> On the basis of this evaluation, which form of intervention is the most efficient?
>
> Although the groupwork participants have achieved a greater reduction of fat consumption, the mass-media campaign is most efficient because it reaches a much greater number of people.

Health promotion is not a technical strategy but a complex means of intervening in people's lives at different levels. The ultimate question of whether or not such activity is justified does not belong to practitioners alone, or managers, or funders, but must involve the whole community. Evaluation is one way of opening up the debate and of ensuring that everyone's voice is heard. Health promoters may be able to demonstrate behaviour change in a desired direction, but this may be at the cost of reduced self-esteem or other undesirable side effects. The sum total of these negative consequences may call into question the benefit of the health promotion intervention.

Definitions of evaluation

Evaluation covers many different activities undertaken with varying degrees of rigour or reflectiveness. At its simplest level, evaluation describes what any competent practitioner does as a matter of course, that is, the process of appraising and assessing work activities. Health promoters

> "... constantly assess the programmes under their control though they may not call the process 'evaluation'. They gauge the rate of progress of a new programme, appraise personal performance, estimate the effectiveness of a particular technique, look at other programmes and compare the results" (Sheiham, 1978).

A cervical cancer screening programme is vigorously advertised and promoted. It results in increased levels of take-up, pre-cancer detection and treatment, but the overall death rate from the disease remains the same. The programme manager thinks it has been a success and that, without the campaign, death rates would have increased. Women participants report increased feelings of disempowerment, depression and anxiety. Has this programme been effective?

This includes the process of informal feedback or more systematic review of health promotion interventions. For example, noting how educational sessions have been received by the audience, or soliciting their comments, or those of peers and colleagues, is part of the evaluation process. Evaluation tends to mean a more formal or systematic activity, where appraisal is linked to original intentions and is fed back into the planning process.

> "Evaluation implies judgement based on careful assessment and critical appraisal of given situations, which should lead to drawing sensible conclusions and making useful proposals for future action" (WHO, 1981, p.9).

Evaluation may be carried out by practitioners or by outside researchers. The latter tend to be larger scale and more ambitious in their remit. There are advantages and drawbacks to each of these options.

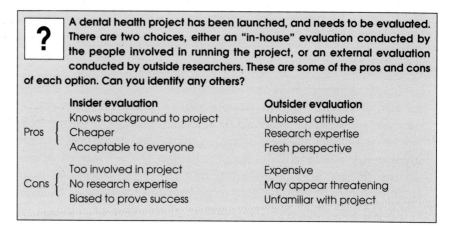

? A dental health project has been launched, and needs to be evaluated. There are two choices, either an "in-house" evaluation conducted by the people involved in running the project, or an external evaluation conducted by outside researchers. These are some of the pros and cons of each option. Can you identify any others?

	Insider evaluation	Outsider evaluation
Pros	Knows background to project Cheaper Acceptable to everyone	Unbiased attitude Research expertise Fresh perspective
Cons	Too involved in project No research expertise Biased to prove success	Expensive May appear threatening Unfamiliar with project

The three Es

Evaluation includes different kinds of activity undertaken for varying reasons. A framework to help identify these differences is given by "the three Es".

1. Efficiency:

The extent to which aims and objectives are attained. This is often measured by comparing results obtained through health promotion with results obtained using other methods, or the different methods used in health promotion may be compared with each other, to see which is best at achieving objectives. Efficiency is sometimes measured by performance appraisal or performance indicators. These techniques are primarily management tools for assessing the efficiency of the workforce.

2. Effectiveness:

The extent to which the objectives set have actually led to desired outcomes. In other words, whether the activity is worthwhile.

3. Economy:

The extent to which outcomes have been achieved economically or in a manner which represents value for money. This can be measured in different ways. Cost analysis compares the costs of a health promotion intervention to the costs of competing activities. Cost effectiveness is a comparison in monetary terms of different methods used to achieve the same outcomes. Cost–benefit analysis is more complicated, and relies on pricing both the inputs and the benefits of a health promotion programme. An attempt is then made to calculate the cost of each benefit. This is known as a cost–benefit ratio. Putting a price on health outcomes or benefits is a very difficult exercise. One approach to this problem is to compare the cost–benefit ratio for a health promotion intervention with the cost–benefit ratio for some other health intervention. It is often assumed that prevention is cheaper than cure and that health promotion saves money, but this is not necessarily the case.

? An effective smoking prevention campaign is associated with the following costs.

Money is saved by:

- Not having to treat people with smoking related diseases on the NHS
- Not having to pay sickness benefit and disability pensions to people with smoking-related diseases
- Increased production in industry because fewer employees are off sick.

Money is lost by:

- Retirement pensions paid to people who live longer
- Unemployment benefits to people in tobacco production and retail industry made unemployed due to fall in demand
- Loss of Government revenue from tobacco taxation.

Overall, do you think this campaign will save money?

? A health promoter sets the objective of increasing knowledge about the transmission of the HIV virus in the expectation that such knowledge will lead to safer sex practices. Review after an educational intervention demonstrates a significant increase in knowledge levels. A follow-up questionnaire reveals that increased knowledge has not led to the desired change in sexual practices.

- Is this intervention efficient?
- Is this intervention effective?

Process, impact and outcome evaluation

Evaluation includes assessments of different kinds of events at varying time periods. A distinction is often made between process, impact and outcome evaluation. Process evaluation (also called formative or illuminative evaluation) is concerned with assessing the process of programme implementation. It addresses participants' perceptions and reactions to health promotion interventions, and identifies the factors which support or impede these activities. Process evaluation employs a wide range of qualitative or "soft" methods. Examples of such methods are interviews, diaries, observations and content analysis of documents. These methods tell us a great deal about that particular programme and the factors responsible for its success or failure, but they are unable to predict what would happen if the programme was replicated in other areas.

Because process evaluation does not use "hard" scientific methods, its findings tend to be more easily dismissed as unrepresentative. However, process evaluation is crucial to health promotion. It is not enough to demonstrate behaviour change or changes in health status. After all, these are constantly changing independently of health promoters. It is also insufficient to assume that implementation is an unproblematic process controlled by policy planners. We need to understand how health promotion interventions are interpreted and responded to by different groups of people, and for this we need process evaluation.

Evaluation of health promotion programmes is usually concerned to identify its effects. The effects of intervention may be divided into two, impact and outcome. Impact refers to immediate effects, whereas outcome refers to more long-term consequences. Impact evaluation tends to be the most popular choice, as it is the easiest to do. Impact evaluation can be built into a programme as the end stage. For example, a health education programme for secondary schools may include as the last session a review of the programme. Students may be invited to identify how they have changed since the programme began and how they think the programme will affect their future behaviour.

Outcome evaluation is more difficult, because it involves an assessment of longer term effects. Using the same example given above, outcome evaluation may be used to determine whether the programme did affect students' behaviour one year later. One way of ascertaining this would be to compare participants' health related behaviour (e.g. smoking, alcohol and exercise) before and after the programme, but there are bound to be changes in students' behaviour over one year, irrespective of any health education programme. So it would be better to compare the students to another group of similar students who did not receive the programme. The second or control group of students is necessary to avoid the danger of attributing all behaviour change to the health education programme and therefore of overestimating its influence.

Outcome evaluation is therefore more complex and costly than impact evaluation. Going back a year later to the same students and getting new information from them will take up time and resources, as will obtaining a matched group of students to use as the control group. However, despite these problems, outcome evaluation is often the preferred evaluation method because it measures sustained changes which have stood the test of time. Results using data on impact or outcome are often expressed numerically, and this again increases credibility. Quantitive or "hard" data are seen as more concrete or factual than the "soft" data used in process evaluation.

> **?**
> **The following include examples of process, impact and outcome evaluation. Which activities are the easiest to do? Which activities are the most useful?**
>
> - Pre- and post-intervention questionnaires testing knowledge levels of participants of a health education programme
> - Take-up levels of a child immunization programme
> - A study of how a district no smoking policy has been implemented
> - Child accident rates 1 year after a 3-month accident prevention campaign
> - A policy review to assess changes in policies affecting health 6 months after the launch of a healthy cities programme
> - Take up of health education literature from leaflet racks in community pharmacies
> - Review of healthy food options available in works canteens 3 months after the launch of a workplace LAYH programme
> - Ongoing assessment of the progress of a local mental health promotion campaign.

Another way of categorizing different types of evaluation is by the type of objective set. Health promotion objectives include knowledge, attitude and behaviour change, as well as change in the environment which may be measured by policy analysis, mass media analysis, changes in legislation, or direct measures of the physical environment. Changes in health status provide another set of objectives, and can include service uptake and use of preventive measures as well as risk factors and morbidity and mortality rates. Although all these factors relate to health, they are quite separate, and there is no necessary connection between, say, increased knowledge and behaviour change. It is therefore inappropriate to evaluate a given objective (e.g. increased exercise rate) by measuring other aspects of an intervention (e.g. number of leaflets taken at a health fair or reported attitude change favouring exercise).

Performance indicators

Performance indicators (PIs) are used in the NHS, and other organizations to measure and monitor activity. PIs are not evaluation measures, but they do measure intermediate or indirect indicators which suggest whether an activity is likely to prove effective. PIs are popular with management because they provide a quantifiable measure of work activity. There is some concern that the use of PIs may lead to health promoters' undertaking activities which can be quantified at the expense of activities which may be more effective but cannot be quantified. However, PIs used in conjunction with target setting do provide a means of monitoring activity, and are part of the evaluation process. The following are examples of PIs used in health promotion.

> ☞ ■ Number of training sessions held and number of participants trained
> ■ Screening take-up rates
> ■ Awareness of mass media health promotion campaign
> ■ Number of leaflets requested and distributed
> ■ Number of workplaces adopting a no smoking policy
> ■ Number of clients offered lifestyle advice and education.

It is important when setting PIs to be realistic about what can be achieved. In particular, care needs to be taken to avoid becoming pressured into adopting unrealistic PIs such as outcomes relating to health status or cost effectiveness. For example, although reduced mortality is often the goal of health promotion, it is unrealistic to use this as a PI. Mortality is affected by many factors and reductions in the mortality rate may take years to become apparent. As we saw earlier, effective health promotion is not necessarily associated with cost cutting.

Pluralistic evaluation

Evaluation is sometimes thought to be an unproblematic part of the health promoter's professional expertise. The assumption is that, faced with a certain set of findings, everyone would agree on their significance or meaning, but this is not necessarily the case. There may also be dispute about which findings are relevant or significant. The example below illustrates these points.

> **?** A road accident prevention programme is launched by a health authority and a local authority. The following groups are involved in the programme:
> ■ Health authority
> ■ Local authority

(cont.)
- Road traffic police
- The community
- The local cycling group
- Staff in the Accident and Emergency Department of the local hospital
- Teachers taking part in the schools programme

Activities include road traffic calming measures, a primary school health education programme, and a free training course for young motocyclists, as well as additional inputs into the national drink–driving campaign. A 6-month interim evaluation found good take up (80%) of the motorcycle training course amongst 16-25 year olds buying motorcycles. Teachers reported good results from the school programme. There was a 10% reduction in the number of drink–drive offences and road traffic accidents. However, out of this reduced number of accidents, the proportion of serious injuries to pedestrians and cyclists increased from 2% to 5%.

- What data would each group be most concerned with?
- Is this a success?
- What do you think the response of each group would be?

Success means different things to different groups of people, or stakeholders, who each have their own agendas and interests (Smith and Cantley, 1985). Different stakeholders have unequal power to impose their evaluation agendas on others. Different groups of people engaged in health promotion interventions will each have invested something but may well be looking for different results. For example, funders of a project may be looking for efficiency or results which can be interpreted as cost effective. Practitioners may be looking for evidence that their way of working is acceptable to clients and achieves the objectives set. Managers may be looking for evidence of increased productivity, measured by performance indicators. Clients may be looking for opportunities to take control over some health-related aspects of their lives.

It is therefore important to be clear at the outset about whose perspectives are being addressed in any evaluation. A starting point is simply to acknowledge that different vested interests are involved and try to identify them. The ideal is to then go on to represent the views of the different stakeholders by collecting data from each group. This process is called pluralistic evaluation (Smith and Cantley, 1985). Using the process of methodological triangulation, which employs a wide range of data sources, an overall picture may be built up. Pluralistic evaluation which takes into account different stakeholder's views is more complete, although the findings may be complex and lack clarity. As Means and Smith (1988, p.27) state:

"... support for pluralistic evaluation requires bravery on the part of the funder. It not only lacks the same level of scientific respectability as the quasi-experimental design but more importantly it is likely to highlight conflicts of interest and perception between all the various groups that have to engage with any programme."

Dilemmas of evaluating health promotion

There are a number of difficulties surrounding attempts to evaluate health promotion. These are both theoretical and practical. In theoretical terms, the many meanings and definitions of the concept "health" mean there is no consensus about how best to evaluate it. For those who subscribe to the medical model of health, data concerning morbidity, disability and mortality are appropriate measures to use for evaluation purposes. For those who adopt a more holistic model of health, a much broader range of measures (including, for example, measures of socio-economic status or the quality of the environment) will be appropriate. For people who prioritize the educational model, measures of knowledge and attitude change will be paramount.

Practical difficulties arise when trying to obtain data and trying to combine different forms of data to provide an overall picture. Some relevant data is already available and accessible, for example, morbidity and mortality data. Other data already exists and may be obtained, for example, policy documents or health surveillance data. However, some data will need to be specially collected and, particularly in areas such as attitude change or empowerment, there are no easy or accepted means of doing this.

Dilemma 1: deciding what to measure

Deciding what to measure to assess the effects of health promotion is not easy. The golden rule must be to measure the objectives set during the planning process. (For more details on programme objectives, see section in Chapter 12 on programme planning). Although this sounds straightforward, in practice it can be difficult, and a surprising number of evaluation studies violate this principle. The objectives set may concern areas where there is a lack of consensus over appropriate measurement. For example, process objectives such as increased multi-agency collaboration or increased community involvement are difficult to measure. To collect relevant data would require a special effort because they are not measured routinely. Change in people's attitudes or beliefs is particularly problematic to measure, and needs specialist input.

A programme may have several different objectives, some of which are easier to measure than others. It then becomes tempting to measure the easiest objectives and extrapolate from these findings. But if the measurements are of different classes of events (e.g. combining behavioural, environmental and attitudinal objectives), it is not legitimate to do this.

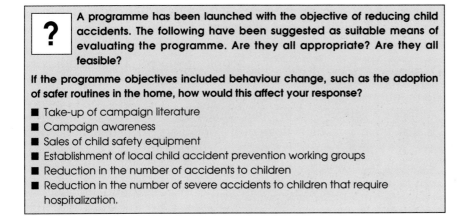

? A programme has been launched with the objective of reducing child accidents. The following have been suggested as suitable means of evaluating the programme. Are they all appropriate? Are they all feasible?

If the programme objectives included behaviour change, such as the adoption of safer routines in the home, how would this affect your response?

- Take-up of campaign literature
- Campaign awareness
- Sales of child safety equipment
- Establishment of local child accident prevention working groups
- Reduction in the number of accidents to children
- Reduction in the number of severe accidents to children that require hospitalization.

Dilemma 2: how to be confident results are due to the health promotion input

Because health promotion is a long-term process and because any situation is constantly changing, it can be difficult to be sure that any changes detected are due to the health promotion input, and not to any other factor. Health-related knowledge, attitudes and behaviour are constantly changing, regardless of health promotion programmes. Societies and environments are also changing in response to many different factors. How can the changes due to health promotion be isolated from everything else? There are two responses to this problem.

The classic scientific method of proof, the experiment, relies on controlling all factors apart from the one being studied. This can best be achieved under laboratory conditions. However, this is clearly impossible and unethical to achieve where people's health is concerned. Instead, the quasi-experimental design is usually the closest that can be achieved. This involves the use of a control group of people who are similar to the group receiving the health promotion input. Factors such as age, gender and social class are all known to affect health. So the control group needs to be matched as closely as possible to the input or experimental group with regard to these factors. Any changes detected in the input group are then compared to those found amongst the control group. Those changes which occur in the input but not the control group can then be attributed to the health promotion programme. Even this degree of scientific rigour is hard to achieve. Most health promotion programmes have spin-off effects and indeed are designed to do so. It is impossible to isolate different groups of people or to ensure that programmes do not "leak" beyond their set boundaries. However, the quasi-experimental design does mean that changes detected in the input group may be ascribed to the health promotion programme with a greater degree of confidence.

It is also possible to use qualitative methods of evaluation. The health promotion programme is treated as a case study and is intensively studied, using a variety of methods if possible. This enables the evaluator to get a detailed picture of how the programme has affected the people involved. These studies are typically small scale and findings are expressed in descriptive rather than numerical terms. Each case study is unique and findings cannot be generalized to other situations. Its strength as a method is that there is a high degree of confidence that identified effects are real and result from the programme. Both the quasi-experimental design and the case study are valid methods which can be used to isolate the effects of health promotion interventions. However, the quasi-experimental design has the higher status and is generally regarded as more respectable and credible than the case study.

Dilemma 3: when to evaluate

Health promotion programmes often have many different effects which will become apparent in different time periods following the intervention. For example, a CHD prevention programme may have the six following effects:

1. Improve people's knowledge of the risk factors for CHD
2. Persuade more people to attend screening clinics
3. Increase media coverage of CHD
4. Prompt various organizations to adopt health policies including CHD prevention
5. Persuade restaurants and cafes to provide healthier meal options
6. Reduce premature mortality rate from CHD.

An immediate post programme evaluation may identify only the first of these effects. An interim (e.g. after 3 months) evaluation may identify the second and third effects. The fourth and fifth effects may only be apparent at a later evaluation, e.g. after 6 months. Six months after the programme, the increased attendance at screening clinics may no longer be discernible and attendance figures have reverted to pre-programme levels. A reduction in the mortality rate may not be discernible for 5 years or more, by which time it will be difficult to attribute it to the health promotion programme. The assessment of the overall success or failure of a programme is therefore influenced by the timing of the evaluation.

Green (1977) has identified five time effects which contribute to the dilemma of short-term versus long-term evaluation. These are as follows:

1. Delay of impact. The effects of a programme may not be immediate but take some time to become apparent. If the desired effect is behaviour change, there may be interim stages such as changes in knowledge or beliefs which need to precede behaviour

change. Immediate evaluation might prove negative, but a longer term evaluation would yield positive results.

2. Decay of impact. Immediate post-programme results reveal positive change has taken place, but this is not sustained, and after some time the situation reverts to how it was pre-programme.

3. Borrowing from the future. Here the programme may speed up a process which was happening anyway. For example, as a general trend people may be taking more exercise. A programme may increase the speed of change and result in real benefits. However, these changes would have happened in the long term without the programme. The effect of the programme is to speed up the process of achieving change.

4. Adjusting for secular trends. Many health promotion programmes concern factors which are already changing in the desired direction, e.g. reduction in smoking. These general trends need to be taken into consideration because only those changes over and above the general trend may be attributed to the programme. If general trends are not taken into account, there is the danger of overestimating the effects of the programme.

5. Backlash effect. Sometimes the positive effects of a programme are not only lost but a contrasting or backlash effect may occur when a programme finishes. This may be due to expectations which have not been met, or cessation of funding or support. Participants may then act in ways contrary to the programme's message. Depending on when evaluation is carried out, findings may be positive or negative.

There is no solution to these problems, but the health promoter should be aware of the issues and try to time their evaluation so as to address those issues most relevant to their particular programme. If possible, evaluation should be carried out at different time periods following a programme but this is often impossible to do.

Dilemma 4: knowing what constitutes success

In this case, there is sufficient knowledge available for an informed assessment of success to take place, but in many other areas of health promotion, this is not the case. We do not know the degree of behaviour change which is likely to occur irrespective of any health promotion programmes, and in general we do not have information comparing different methods or strategies. So if specific objectives are set, they are often a "shot in the dark", and may be either too ambitious or too modest. For example, it has been argued that the targets set in the *Health of the Nation* take no account of local variations. Consequently, in some areas, some of

---

A smoking cessation programme is launched which includes clinics for those wishing to give up smoking. A clinic run by a health promoter attracts 20 clients who attend all six sessions. At a 6-month evaluation, 25% participants have stopped smoking. Is this a success?
The health promoter may be pleased with these results. People attend clinics often as a last resort, and 6 months is a reasonable time period to assess long-term behaviour change. However, their manager may point out that 20% is an average success rate for people trying to quit regardless of what methods are used. Clinics are time consuming and 20 people is not a large group. Twenty-five per cent quitters is five people, four of whom might have quit using other less intensive or expensive methods. So one additional ex-smoker might be the result of the smoking cessation clinic.

the targets are too modest, and on current trends could be expected to be met with no additional input. Conversely, some targets are too ambitious for other areas and are very unlikely to be met (Mihill, 1992).

Dilemma 5: is evaluation worth the effort?

In the light of all the problems identified above, and given the fact that evaluation consumes limited resources, is evaluation worth the effort? Assessing the value of one's work is an important aspect of being a reflective practitioner. We have already discussed the role of performance indicators in monitoring and evaluating one's work. Deciding when a more formal or complete evaluation should be undertaken is not easy.

Ongoing routine work which is based on previously demonstrated effectiveness or efficiency is probably not worthwhile evaluating in depth. However, new or pilot interventions do warrant a more thorough-going evaluation because, without evidence of their effectiveness or efficiency, it is difficult to argue that they should become established work practices. Other criteria that can be used to determine if evaluation is worth the effort relate to how well it can be done. If it will be impossible to obtain co-operation from the different groups involved in the activity, it is probably not worthwhile trying to evaluate. If evaluation has not been considered at the outset but is tacked on as an "afterthought", the chances are it will be so partial and biased as to be not worth the effort.

Evaluation is only worthwhile if it will make a difference. This means that the results of the evaluation need to be interpreted and fed back to the relevant audiences in an accessible form. All too often, evaluations are buried in inappropriate formats. Work reports may go no further than the manager, or academic studies full of jargon may be published in little-known journals.

Results of evaluation studies will be relevant to many different groups and it may be necessary to reproduce findings in different ways in order to reach all these groups.

 A district nurse has evaluated her health promotion activities. These include opportunistic one-to-one counselling and education, setting up a carers' support group, producing information leaflets on coping with dementia, and health surveys of people aged 75 and over.

How could she make her findings known to her clients, her manager, her nursing colleagues, and other health and welfare workers?

Conclusion

Evaluation contributes to the accountability and development of health promotion practice, and so is an important aspect of the health promoter's work. There are often pressures to adopt unrealistic measures of success, such as reduced mortality rates or demonstrable cost benefits. Most health promoters are engaged in more modest activities which seek to achieve changes in behaviour, knowledge, attitudes, service take-up or the policy process. These are more appropriate outcomes to use for evaluation purposes.

Evaluation is a practical activity which feeds into the theoretical debate about the nature and purpose of health promotion. This debate cannot be confined to professionals, or those who hold managerial or financial power. It must include the public, those who are the targets of health promotion activity. This is why pluralistic evaluation, which enables participants to have a voice in determining effectiveness, is so important. Evaluation can be thought of as a bridge linking health promoters to others, including clients, funders, managers and colleagues.

Evaluation is not a simple activity and it consumes resources which might otherwise be spent on doing health promotion. The decision about whether, when and how to evaluate is therefore important. The question of evaluation should be considered at the outset of any planned health promotion intervention. If it is to be done, it should be done in the best possible way. If this is not feasible, then it is better to admit the impossible, and not attempt to evaluate. Ongoing monitoring may be the best one can do. This is acceptable, but there is a distinction between routine monitoring of activities through the use of performance indicators and a more thorough-going evaluation. It is important not to confuse the two and to be clear about which it is you are doing.

The following have been suggested as guidelines for good practice in evaluation.

Which do you think should be included in a checklist "Criteria to be met if undertaking evaluation"? Are there any other guidelines you would wish to add?

- Evaluate early on before vested interests have had time to solidify
- Evaluate only if it will make a difference
- Evaluate only when it is appropriate
- Evaluate only when you can include the perceptions of different groups, e.g. only when you can do a pluralistic evaluation
- Publicize the results of evaluation widely in relevant formats
- Evaluate only when there is a chance of scientific accuracy
- If you can't meet these criteria, don't evaluate.

Questions for further discussion

- ■ What factors would influence your decision about whether to evaluate a particular health promotion activity?
- ■ What factors would you wish to consider when evaluating a health promotion intervention?

Summary

This chapter has looked at why health promotion needs to be evaluated and examined the definition of evaluation, using the three Es as a checklist. Different kinds of evaluation have been identified, including process, impact and outcome evaluation. The notion of stakeholders, leading to the necessity for pluralistic evaluation, has been discussed. Finally, five central dilemmas in the practice of evaluation have been examined.

Further reading

Aggleton P, Moody D and Young A (1992) *Evaluating HIV/AIDS Health Promotion*, London, HEA.

A detailed and user-friendly guide, with lots of suggestions and exercises. Although the book is concerned with HIV/AIDS, the ideas could be applied to other areas of health promotion work.

Means R and Smith R (1988) "Implementing a pluralistic approach to evaluation in health education", *Policy and Politics*, **16**, 17–28.

A good example of pluralistic evaluation, including a discussion of its advantages and disadvantages in practice.

Tones K, Tilford S and Robinson Y (1990) *Health Education: Effectiveness and Efficiency*, London, Chapman & Hall.

A detailed look at how success in health education is measured in different settings.

World Health Organisation (1981) *Health Programme Evaluation: Guiding Principles*, Geneva, WHO.

A short and practical guide to the principles underlying evaluation. It outlines a staged process for evaluating health promotion programmes.

References

Bell J, Billington DR, Macdonald M, Drummond N and Thompson G (1985) *Annotated Bibliography of Health Education Research Completed in Britain from 1948–1978 and 1979–1983*, Edinburgh, Scottish Health Education Group.

Cochrane AL (1972) *Effectiveness and Efficiency*, Nuffield Provincial Hospitals Trust.

Gatherer A, Parfit J, Porter E and Vessey M (1979) *Is Health Education Effective?* London, Health Education Council.

Green L (1977) "Education and measurement: some dilemmas for health education", *American Journal of Public Health*, **67**, 155–162.

Green LW and Lewis FM (1986) *Measurement and Evaluation in Health Education and Health Promotion*, Mountain View, California, Mayfield.

Means R and Smith R (1988) "Implementing a pluralistic approach to evaluation in health education", *Policy and Politics*, **16**, 17–28.

Mihill C (1992) "Strategy for improvement or window dressing?", *The Guardian*, 9/7/1992.

Sheiham A (1978) "Evaluating health education programmes", *Health Education Journal*, **37**, 127–131.

Smith G and Cantley C (1985) *Assessing Health Care: A Study in Organisational Evaluation*, Milton Keynes, Open University Press.

Tones K, Tilford S and Robinson Y (1990) *Health Education: Effectiveness and Efficiency.* London, Chapman & Hall.

World Health Organisation (1981) *Health Programme Evaluation: Guiding Principles*, Geneva, WHO.

Subject index